Questions & Answers About Overactive Bladder
Second Edition

Pamela Ellsworth, MD
Division of Urology
Brown University
Providence, RI

Alan J. Wein, MD, PhD (Hon.)
Chief, Division of Urology
University of Pennsylvania Health Systems
Philadelphia, PA

JONES AND BARTLETT PUBLISHERS
Sudbury, Massachusetts
BOSTON   TORONTO   LONDON   SINGAPORE

World Headquarters
Jones and Bartlett Publishers
40 Tall Pine Drive
Sudbury, MA 01776
978-443-5000
info@jbpub.com
www.jbpub.com

Jones and Bartlett Publishers
Canada
6339 Ormindale Way
Mississauga, Ontario L5V 1J2
Canada

Jones and Bartlett Publishers
International
Barb House, Barb Mews
London W6 7PA
United Kingdom

Jones and Bartlett's books and products are available through most bookstores and online booksellers.
To contact Jones and Bartlett Publishers directly, call 800-832-0034, fax 978-443-8000, or visit our
website www.jbpub.com.

Substantial discounts on bulk quantities of Jones and Bartlett's publications are available to
corporations, professional associations, and other qualified organizations. For details and specific
discount information, contact the special sales department at Jones and Bartlett via the above
contact information or send an email to specialsales@jbpub.com.

The authors, editor, and publisher have made every effort to provide accurate information. However,
they are not responsible for errors, omissions, or for any outcomes related to the use of the contents of
this book and take no responsibility for the use of the products and procedures described. Treatments
and side effects described in this book may not be applicable to all people; likewise, some people may
require a dose or experience a side effect that is not described herein. Drugs and medical devices are discussed that may have limited availability controlled by the Food and Drug Administration (FDA) for
use only in a research study or clinical trial. Research, clinical practice, and government regulations
often change the accepted standard in this field. When consideration is being given to use of any drug
in the clinical setting, the healthcare provider or reader is responsible for determining FDA status of the
drug, reading the package insert, and reviewing prescribing information for the most up-to-date recommendations on dose, precautions, and contraindications, and determining the appropriate usage for the
product. This is especially important in the case of drugs that are new or seldom used.

Production Credits
Executive Publisher: Christopher Davis
Production Editor: Daniel Stone
Sr. Editorial Assistant: Jessica Acox
Marketing Manager: Ilana Goddess
V.P., Manufacturing and Inventory Control: Therese Connell
Composition: Auburn Associates, Inc.
Printing and Binding: Malloy, Inc.
Cover Design: Carolyn Downer
Cover Printing: Malloy, Inc.

Cover Image Credits
Upper Left: © Monkey Business Images/ShutterStock, Inc.; Upper Right: © Monkey Business
Images/ShutterStock, Inc.; Bottom Left: © absolut/ShutterStock, Inc.; Bottom Right:
© dundanim/ShutterStock, Inc.

Library of Congress Cataloging-in-Publication Data
Ellsworth, Pamela.
    Questions & answers about overactive bladder / Pamela Ellsworth, Alan J. Wein.—2nd ed.
        p. cm.
    Includes bibliographical references and index.
    ISBN-13: 978-0-7637-7198-0 (alk. paper)
    ISBN-10: 0-7637-7198-8 (alk. paper)
    1. Urinary incontinence—Popular works. 2. Urinary incontinence—Miscellanea. 3. Bladder—
Popular works. 4. Bladder—Miscellanea. I. Wein, Alan J. II. Title. III. Title: Questions and
answers about overactive bladder.
    RC921.I5E45 2009
    616.6'2—dc22
                                                                                    2009007142
6048

Printed in the United States of America
13 12 11 10 09   10 9 8 7 6 5 4 3 2 1

Contents

Preface   **v**

Part 1: The Basics   **1**

Questions 1-8 provide fundamental information about the bladder and incontinence, including:

- What is the bladder, and what does it do?
- What are normal voiding habits?
- What problems can occur with bladder function?

Part 2: Diagnosis of Overactive Bladder   **17**

Questions 9-31 discuss the identification of incontinence due to overactive bladder:

- What is overactive bladder?
- What is the natural history of overactive bladder? Is it permanent? Can it resolve
  or does it come and go?
- What causes OAB?

Part 3: Treatment of Overactive Bladder   **51**

Questions 32-80 describe nonsurgical, minimally invasive, and surgical options for
treatment of overactive bladder:

- What are the options for treating OAB?
- What are pelvic floor muscle exercises (Kegel exercises)?
- What is neuromodulation/sacral nerve stimulation?
- What is bladder augmentation?

Glossary   **121**
Index   **129**

Overactive bladder (OAB) is a term used to describe the symptom complex of urgency; and a sudden, compelling desire to urinate that is difficult to postpone, often associated with urinary frequency (urinating more than 8 times in 24 hours), nocturia (getting up from sleep because of the need to urinate), and, in many, urgency incontinence (leaking urine because of the inability to get to the bathroom in time). Overactive bladder (OAB) and urinary incontinence affect over 30 million Americans, male and female. The risk of developing overactive bladder increases with age in both males and females. Overall one-third of people with OAB have some urinary incontinence. This is more common in women than in men. Urinary incontinence is responsible for nearly 50% of nursing home admissions. Overactive bladder is associated with a significant negative impact on quality of life and increases the risk of urinary tract infections, skin irritation, and, in elderly females, an increased risk of falls and fractures. The economic impact of overactive bladder is huge; continence supplies, such as diapers and pads, are only a portion of the healthcare dollars spent on this condition.

Despite the high prevalence, the significant effects on quality of life, the associated medical morbidities, and the financial impact of overactive bladder and urgency incontinence, this condition remains largely under-diagnosed and untreated. Often, it takes several years before patients seek evaluation and treatment. Why is this the case? Unfortunately, there are several barriers to the identification and treatment of overactive bladder, both on the part of the patient and the physician. OAB sufferers may believe that (1) the condition is an inevitable part of aging, which is an incorrect assumption; (2) the condition is too embarrassing to discuss with anyone, including the physician; (3) the symptoms are "minor" compared to those of their friends/family with "life-threatening" illnesses and therefore not deserving of attention; (4) there are no medical therapies that can treat the condition; and (5) they may need to undergo expensive and invasive testing to accurately diagnose their problem. Some individuals may bring the subject up with their doctors. This, however, is often not the case initially and leads to a delay in diagnosis and treatment. Furthermore, even if the subject is addressed, only a small percentage of patients are actually evaluated and treated. The evaluation and management of overactive bladder continues to evolve as knowledge is gained regarding the causes of overactive bladder, and new therapies, medical and minimally invasive, are being investigated for use in treating overactive bladder. In the past 5 to 10 years the number of medications and other therapies used for the treatment of overactive bladder has almost tripled.

Many of the limitations in the evaluation and management of overactive bladder are the result of inadequate knowledge and awareness. It is our sincere hope that this book provides knowledge to empower OAB sufferers to seek help and to be actively involved in their management plan so that their quality of life and medical health may be improved. If we can touch the lives of even a few OAB sufferers, we will have achieved our goal. Read on and find out how you can take back your control. Control your bladder—do not let it control you.

PART ONE

The Basics

What is the bladder, and what does it do?

What are normal voiding habits?

What problems can occur with bladder function?

More ...

1. What is the bladder, and what does it do?

The bladder is a hollow organ shaped like a sphere that is specially designed to accomplish two tasks. It stores urine at low pressures, and when full, it empties urine. For the bladder to accomplish these tasks, it must be able to stretch and accommodate increasing amounts of fluid (urine). This prevents any increases in bladder pressure or rupture of the bladder. This ability of the bladder to stretch is a result of the elastic and fibrous tissue between the lining of the bladder (**urothelium**) and the bladder muscle (**detrusor**). At a certain point, the bladder muscle must be able to contract strongly and efficiently so that urine can be forced out of the organ and the bladder completely emptied of fluid.

Infants have very little storage because the bladder fills and empties frequently. As an infant matures into a toddler and small child, the lines of communication between the bladder and brain mature, allowing the brain to control the bladder. Thus, when a child is "potty trained," he or she has the ability to hold urine and then voluntarily empty the bladder at a socially acceptable time. During childhood development the bladder grows with the rest of the body. It continues to increase in size until adolescence, when an adult size bladder is achieved. A normal adult bladder capacity is around 10 to 15 ounces (400 cc [cubic centimeters]).

The kidneys produce urine constantly. Urine passes from each kidney down the **ureter**, which is a long, thin, hollow tubular structure, and drains into the bladder (see **Figure 1**).

Urothelium

The innermost lining layer of the urinary tract.

Detrusor

Another name given to the muscle which comprises the bladder contractile mechanism. Coordinated contraction of the detrusor and opening of the bladder outlet allows for normal urination.

Ureter

A long, thin, hollow tubular structure connecting the kidneys to the bladder. The ureter propels urine from the kidneys into the bladder.

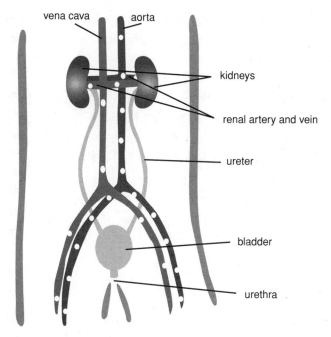

vena cava   aorta

kidneys

renal artery and vein

ureter

bladder

urethra

Figure 1   Anatomy of the GU tract

The wall of the ureter has muscle fibers in it that alternately contract and relax, propelling urine down the ureter into the bladder. This contraction of the ureter, along with gravity, helps ensure that urine moves from the kidney into the bladder. If the bladder pressure is high, the ureter may be unable to push urine into the bladder and a backup of urine, called **stasis,** may result within the ureter and ultimately the kidney. Therefore, while the bladder is storing urine, it also must exhibit compliance, that is, it must be able to store urine at a low pressure until capacity is reached—in other words, it is "full". When the bladder is full, the muscle contracts, raising the bladder pressure, which leads to the expulsion of urine.

Bladder emptying in the toilet-trained individual is under voluntary control. During bladder filling, and

Stasis

A circumstance in which high pressure in the bladder causes a backup of urine within the ureter and eventually the kidney. Stasis of urine may also occur in the bladder if there is decreased bladder contractility or bladder outlet obstruction.

3

Bladder outlet

Area where the bladder joins the urethra.

Urethra

Canal leading from the bladder to the body's skin to discharge urine externally. In the female, it is ~4cm long and opens in the perineum between the clitoris and vaginal opening; in the male it is ~20cm long and opens in the glans penis.

Continence

Ability to retain urine and/or feces until a proper time for their discharge.

Urethral sphincter

A group of muscles that closes the urethra when contracted.

Central nervous system

Found in the brain and spinal cord; responsible for starting or preventing urination.

Peripheral nervous system

Nerves in the body other than in the brain and spinal cord.

urine storage, the **bladder outlet**, which is the area where the bladder joins the **urethra**, remains closed (see **Figure 2**).

This maintains **continence** (no urine leakage) during bladder filling and storage. During voiding (emptying) there is coordination between the bladder and the urethra such that as the bladder contracts the bladder outlet opens, allowing for the release of urine through the bladder outlet into the urethra. The **urethral sphincter,** a group of muscles that closes the urethra when contracted, also relaxes during voiding to allow for the passage of urine through the entire urethra. The nervous system is the ultimate control system for urination.

The nervous system is composed of two parts: the **central nervous system** (brain and spinal cord) and the **peripheral nervous system** (nerves found outside

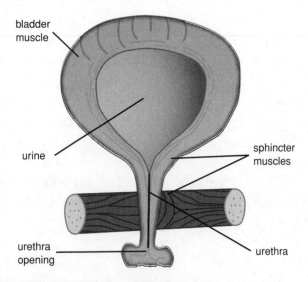

Bladder and Sphincter Muscles (Female)

bladder muscle

urine

sphincter muscles

urethra opening

urethra

Figure 2   Bladder and bladder outlet in the woman
National Institute of Diabetes and Digestive and Kidney Diseases, National Institutes of Health.

of the central nervous system). Bioelectrical signals are constantly flowing from one nerve to another, telling cells in the body what to do and when to do it. Some of these signals are consciously given—when you want to move an arm, for example—and other signals are given without you knowing about them. These unconscious signals drive most of the complicated bodily functions, such as blood flow, heart rate, etc.

The nervous system is responsible for starting or preventing urination and for the coordination of bladder contraction and urethral relaxation during normal voiding. The nerves which control bladder function are primarily the pelvic and hypogastric nerves. Activation of the pelvic nerve leads to contraction of the bladder (see **Figure 3**). Signals from the hypogastric nerve (see **Figure 4**) act to promote urine storage in the bladder.

**Contractile Innervation
and Receptors**

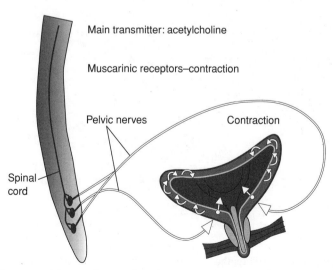

Figure 3   Pelvic nerve innervation of the bladder

The pudendal nerve controls contraction and relaxation of the main urethral sphincter in the bladder outlet. Relaxation allows urine to pass out of the bladder and through the urethra (see Figure 4).

When the pelvic nerves are stimulated, there is a release of a chemical, a neurotransmitter called **acetylcholine**, from the end of the nerve. Acetylcholine then attaches to specialized areas in the bladder muscle wall, called receptors, like a baseball caught by a glove, and this combination activates a series of events which stimulates the bladder muscle to contract. These receptors in the bladder for acetylcholine are called **muscarinic receptors**. There are a total of five different types of muscarinic receptors located throughout the body. In the bladder, there are primarily two identified categories of muscarinic receptors, termed M2 and M3. Although the majority of the muscarinic receptors in the bladder are M2 receptors, it appears that the receptor primarily responsible for bladder contraction is the M3 receptor. M2 receptors may have a role in bladder contraction in certain abnormal conditions. The sym-

Acetylcholine

The chemical which is released from the pelvic nerves and causes contraction of the bladder muscle cells by attaching to a specialized component (receptor) on the bladder muscle cell membrane.

Muscarinic receptor

A membrane-bound protein that contains a recognition site for acetylcholine; combination of acetylcholine with the receptor initiates a physiologic change (i.e., slowing of the heart rate, increased glandular activity, and stimulation of smooth muscle contractions).

Innervation of the Lower Urinary Tract (LUT)

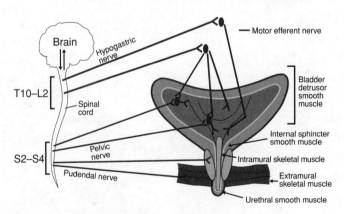

Figure 4 Innervation of the lower urinary tract
Adapted from Wein AJ. *Exp Opin Invest Drugs*. 2001:10:65-83.

The Basics

pathetic nervous system helps the bladder to store urine by causing the bladder muscle to relax. Storage of urine is also aided by the closure of the bladder neck and contraction of the urethral sphincter muscle.

Usually, there is no sensation of bladder fullness until the bladder is about one quarter to one third full. Once the bladder has filled to about half of its capacity, the first sensation of bladder fullness reaches the central nervous system in the brain. At this time, there is some awareness of the need to **urinate**, but one can voluntarily suppress this. An example of this is when you are driving in the car and you feel the urge to urinate, but there are no restrooms around you. Normally, you can suppress this urge and hold onto the urine until you can locate a restroom. At about three-quarters' capacity there is a stronger desire to urinate.

Urinate
To excrete urine.

2. What are normal voiding habits?

It is hard to say what "normal voiding habits" are, because voiding frequency is dependent on fluid intake, the types of fluids that you drink, the medications that you take, and the situations that you are in. Typically, it is thought that the average adult voids roughly every 3 to 4 hours while awake and can sleep through the night without having to urinate. Individuals who void more than eight times per day are said to have **urinary frequency**, and those who get up at night because they need to urinate have **nocturia.** Remember, however, that if you drink six cups of coffee in the morning, you will need to void frequently due to the diuretic effect of the fluid plus the caffeine. Similarly, if you drink three quarts of fluid per day, you will need

Urinary frequency
Having to void more than eight times per day with normal intake of fluids.

Nocturia
Having to wake from sleep at night to urinate after a day of normal fluid intake; causes include increased urine production at night, incomplete bladder emptying, sleep problems, or overactive bladder.

to urinate more than eight times in the day. Individuals who take diuretics, sometimes called "water pills," may also experience urinary frequency because of the increased urine volume that the medication produces. Some of these medications exert most of their actions within the space of a few hours and so cause an increase in urinary frequency only during that time.

Urinary incontinence

Involuntary loss of urine. May be the result of an overactive bladder, stress incontinence, functional incontinence, or other causes.

Small capacity bladder

Organ cannot hold much urine because of fibrosis or scarring or neurologic causes; the bladder loses its elasticity so the individual must urinate more frequently.

Overactive bladder

A symptom complex characterized by urgency, with or without urgency urinary incontinence, usually with frequency and nocturia often associated with involuntary contractions of the bladder (detrusor overactivity).

3. What problems can occur with bladder function?

The urinary bladder has two main functions: one is to fill with and store urine at a low pressure and the other is to expel urine. Problems with bladder function may relate to either of these two functions or both.

Storage problems include **urinary incontinence** (leakage), **small capacity bladder**, and an **overactive bladder**. Emptying problems include a bladder that does not contract in a normal fashion, or at all, and obstruction in the bladder outlet (the passage through which the urine flows after leaving the bladder).

Storage Problems

A small capacity bladder is one that does not hold much urine. This may be related to fibrosis or scarring within the bladder or from neurologic causes (a problem in the nerves, the spinal cord, or the brain). In this situation, the bladder loses its ability to stretch so it cannot hold the expected amount of urine. With this condition, one tends to void more frequently.

The term overactive bladder (OAB) refers to a set of storage symptoms. The primary symptom of overactive bladder is urgency. Urgency is a sudden compelling desire to void that is difficult to defer. It is generally associated with the fear of leaking urine. Urgency is different than the urge to void, which is a normal sensation and gets stronger if you hold off voiding. Urgency comes on suddenly and typically causes one to stop activities and rush to the bathroom. Urgency may be associated with urine leakage, called urgency urinary incontinence or urge urinary incontinence. Other symptoms of overactive bladder usually include urinary frequency (voiding eight or more times per day) and nocturia (awakening one or more times per night to urinate). These symptoms may be related to involuntary contractions of the bladder (termed detrusor overactivity), increased or inappropriate nerve impulses from the bladder to the brain, or an inability of the brain to properly interpret and control the impulses that are sent to it.

A **poorly compliant bladder** refers to a bladder in which the pressure rises gradually with filling by urine but at a higher rate than normal, resulting in a higher pressure than normal at a particular volume. The elevated bladder pressure can cause poor emptying of the kidneys, a backup of urine in the kidneys, and, eventually, kidney damage.

Poorly compliant bladder

Holds urine at higher than normal bladder pressures, causing poor emptying of the kidneys, a backup of urine in the kidneys, and eventually kidney damage.

Emptying Problems

Normal bladder contractility is important in emptying of the bladder. If there is an element of obstruction or blockage to the outflow of urine from the bladder (such as with prostate enlargement), scar tissue causing narrowed areas at the bladder neck or in the urethra (contractures or strictures), or medications that increase the tone of the urethral musculature, the bladder must

Poor contractility

A situation in which the bladder cannot generate and/or sustain a contraction capable of completely emptying it of urine.

Congenital anomalies

Existing at birth; refers to physical traits, conditions, diseases, abnormalities, or malformations, etc., which may be either hereditary or the result of an influence occurring during gestation up to the moment of birth.

Acontractile bladder

A bladder that does not contract.

Urinary retention, acute

The inability to urinate on one's own.

be able to generate a higher pressure than normal to overcome the obstruction. In certain cases there may be **poor contractility** of the bladder, meaning that the bladder muscle cannot generate a strong enough squeeze (contraction) and/or sustain the contraction to completely empty the bladder. Poor bladder contractility may result from injury to the nerves supplying the bladder, such as after an operation in the pelvis or in spinal cord injury, **congenital anomalies** (abnormalities that are present at birth), such as spina bifida (myelomeningocele), chronic overdistention of the bladder, severe long-term outlet obstruction, or medications that reduce bladder contractility. Poor contractility of the bladder may lead to increasing amounts of urine left behind in the bladder after voiding. This "post-void residual" urine may lead to urinary tract infections, bladder stones, further distention of the bladder, worsening of the bladder function, and/or elevated bladder pressures that cause dilation of the ureters and kidneys and possible damage to the kidneys.

An **acontractile bladder** is one that does not contract. This may occur suddenly with no prior history of trouble with urination or it may be part of a slowly progressive problem. The individual may or may not feel an urge to urinate and will not be able to urinate. It is very important to treat **urinary retention** (the inability to urinate at all) immediately to prevent kidney (renal) damage.

4. Is there an age when one is most at risk for urinary incontinence?

The prevalence of urinary incontinence, defined as involuntary leakage of urine or the leakage of urine from the urinary tract without the owner's permission, increases with age for both males and females. Unfortunately, because urinary incontinence is so common in older women, it is sometimes misperceived as a normal and inevitable part of aging. This is not true!

In women, the prevalence of urinary incontinence in some amount in the general population is 20% to 30% for young adults, 30% to 40% for middle-aged women, and 30% to 50% for elderly women.

In males, the prevalence of urinary incontinence is about 3% to 11% overall, with **urge (urgency) incontinence** accounting for 40% to 80% of the patients. **Stress incontinence** is uncommon in males, accounting for less than 10% of cases, and is usually related to prior pelvic or prostate surgery, pelvic trauma, or a neurological injury.

Remember that even though the risk of developing an overactive bladder increases with age, it is not a "normal expected part of aging" and, more importantly, it can be treated.

5. Are there other causes of urinary incontinence besides urgency incontinence?

Indeed, there are several other types of urinary incontinence. "Stress" urinary incontinence is the involuntary loss of urine on effort or exertion, such as during heavy lifting, or on sneezing or coughing. **Mixed urinary incontinence** is the complaint of involuntary leakage associated with urgency and also with exertion, effort, sneezing, or coughing. **Functional incontinence**

The Basics

Urge (urgency) incontinence

Unintended leakage or loss of urine into clothing as a result of detrusor overactivity.

Stress incontinence

Also known as genuine stress urinary incontinence (GSUI), involuntary loss of bladder control during periods of increased abdominal pressure such as coughing, laughing, heavy lifting, or straining.

Mixed urinary incontinence

Involuntary leakage of urine associated with urgency as well as with exertion, effort, sneezing, or coughing. The combination of urgency incontinence and stress urinary incontinence.

Functional incontinence

A situation in which the bladder, urethra, and pelvic floor muscles are functioning properly, but physical or mental function interferes with one's ability to independently get to the bathroom on time.

is a situation in which the bladder, urethra, and pelvic floor muscles are functioning, but abnormal physical or mental function interferes with one's ability to independently get to the bathroom in time. Think of someone whose ability to walk or move about is limited or who has dementia or mental retardation. Chronic retention may lead to leakage of urine when the bladder is over-distended (expanded beyond its elastic capacity); this is called overflow incontinence. This usually is the result of obstruction to the outflow of urine due to prostate enlargement in men but may also result from neurologic diseases, poor bladder muscle function, or as a side effect of medications. Incontinence may be caused by illness or medications that temporarily cause functional incontinence

6. How can I tell the difference between incontinence associated with an overactive bladder (urge or urgency incontinence) and stress incontinence?

A review of symptoms and physical examination will allow you and your healthcare provider to identify the cause of your urinary leakage. Some women will have both stress and urgency incontinence, so there may be more than one cause for urine leakage. An assessment of the presence or absence of the following symptoms will help to identify the cause of urine leakage (see **Table 1**).

Physical examination of the incontinent female includes an examination of the **perineum**. During this part of the examination, you will be asked to strain/bear down (Valsalva maneuver) and cough while the physician

Perineum

Area between the thighs extending from the tail bone (coccyx) to the pubis (between the vulva and anus in the female and scrotum and anus in the male) and lying below the pelvic diaphragm.

Table 1 Symptoms found in overactive bladder and stress incontinence

Symptoms	Overactive Bladder	Stress Incontinence
Urgency	Yes	No
Frequency with urgency	Yes	No
Leakage with physical activity (cough, laugh, sneeze)	No	Yes
Amount of urine leaked with each episode	Usually large, if present	Usually small
Ability to reach toilet in time following an urge to void	No or just barely	Yes
Need to wake up at night to urinate	Often yes	Not often

Radical prostatectomy

Removal of the entire prostate, a procedure performed for prostate cancer.

Transurethral resection

Removal of the central portion of the prostate to make the outlet wider and reduce obstruction.

Urodynamic study

A test which evaluates the ability of the bladder to fill with and store urine as well as to empty; the function of the outlet is to remain closed during bladder filling and to stay open during bladder emptying; study determines the presence or absence of outlet obstruction.

watches for abnormal movement of the urethra (hyper-mobility) and simultaneous leakage of urine. The presence of leakage with a Valsalva maneuver (straining) indicates stress urinary incontinence. Men rarely develop stress incontinence except occasionally after prostate surgery, such as a **radical prostatectomy** for prostate cancer or a **transurethral resection** or other procedure for benign enlargement of the prostate.

Less commonly, the physician may perform a **urodynamic study** as an investigative tool to determine the etiology of your urinary symptoms (see Question 30). When an overactive bladder is present, the urodynamic study will often show contractions of the bladder which occur without the owner's permission at a time when the bladder muscle should be relaxed.

The Basics

7. I have overactive bladder symptoms and urgency incontinence, but I also leak when I cough, laugh, or sneeze. Is it possible to have both overactive bladder with urgency incontinence and stress incontinence?

It is possible to have both overactive bladder and urgency incontinence as well as stress incontinence (see **Figure 5**).

The presence of both stress incontinence and urgency incontinence is called mixed incontinence. Both are treatable. It is important that you discuss the symptoms of both with your healthcare provider. Depending on the severity of your symptoms, and which is more bothersome—the overactive bladder symptoms or the stress incontinence—your provider may elect to treat one of these conditions first and hold off on

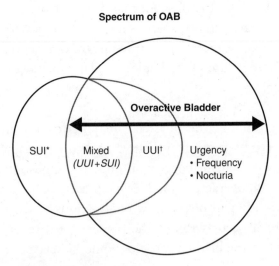

Spectrum of OAB

Figure 5 Spectrum of OAB/incontinence
*SUI = stress urinary incontinence
†UUI = urgency urinary incontinence

treating the other conditions until a satisfactory result has been obtained with the first. Sometimes successful treatment of one can benefit the other.

8. What is interstitial cystitis or painful bladder? How do I tell whether I have this or overactive bladder?

Interstitial cystitis is the name originally given to a condition characterized by pain or discomfort in the bladder and/or pelvic area usually related moreso to bladder filling, and subsiding somewhat or completely with emptying, and associated with urinary frequency. It is more common in woman than in men. Approximately 1.3 million Americans have interstitial cystitis and more than 1 million are female. The symptoms of interstitial cystitis may vary among people; even the same person can have different symptoms at different times. The pain and discomfort can vary from a mild discomfort, pressure or tenderness in the bladder and pelvic area, to significant pain. Although this was originally called interstitial cystitis, it is often not associated with inflammation. The tendency now is to call this entity bladder pain syndrome or painful bladder syndrome. However, in some individuals the pain may seem to be primarily in the urethra, vagina, or elsewhere in the pelvis. Patients with interstitial cystitis/painful bladder syndrome may usually complain of urgency and/or frequency but rarely of incontinence. Their feeling of urgency, however, is not associated with a fear of leaking urine but rather with pain which can often be lessened by voiding and can often be made worse by further bladder filling. Patients may describe an improvement in the discomfort when they urinate. Some women will note that the symptoms are worse during menstruation. Some women will also note pain with intercourse (dyspareunia).

The symptoms of bladder pain syndrome/interstitial cystitis probably arise from a variety of conditions, not just one. The diagnosis is usually one of exclusion meaning ruling out other conditions that may cause similar symptoms, such as urinary tract infections, overactive bladder, bladder cancer, and, in men, inflammation/ infection of the prostate. The diagnosis is usually based on the association of pain with the symptoms, which is not typically present in patients with overactive bladder.

In some individuals with symptoms of interstitial cystitis, a cystoscopy (a look into the bladder with a special instrument that looks like a small telescope) may be helpful. Findings on cystoscopy such as small pinpoint areas of bleeding in the bladder lining (glomerulations), or Hunner's ulcers, small tears in the bladder lining, are felt to be indicative of what was originally called interstitial cystitis. The cystoscopy is performed under anesthesia as it is often too painful to do in the office. At the time of the cystoscopy, the bladder is filled with a sterile fluid to determine how much fluid the bladder holds. Many people with bladder pain syndrome/interstitial cystitis have bladders that only hold onto only a small amount of fluid. Filling of the bladder, to a maximum pressure called hydrodistention, may temporarily improve the symptoms of interstitial cystitis/ painful bladder syndrome.

PART TWO

Diagnosis of Overactive Bladder

What is overactive bladder?

What is the natural history of overactive bladder?
Is it permanent? Can it resolve or
does it come and go?

What causes OAB?

More . . .

9. What is overactive bladder?

Overactive bladder (OAB) symptoms suggest the presence of involuntary bladder contractions, contractions which are abnormal and occur without the owner's permission, also known as detrusor overactivity (DO). Typically during bladder filling and storage, the bladder muscle remains relaxed to hold urine and contracts only at the time of urination. DO may be felt as a need to urinate or, if the contraction is strong enough or the pelvic floor muscles weakened, there may be loss of urine. If DO occurs frequently, the result is urinary frequency. OAB may also be the result of increased activity in the "afferent or sensory nerves." The afferent nerves send messages from the bladder regarding bladder filling, stretch, and pain to the brain. It is thought that increased activity in these nerves and/or inability of the brain to control or properly interpret this activity may lead to some of the symptoms of OAB, such as urgency (see **Figure 6**).

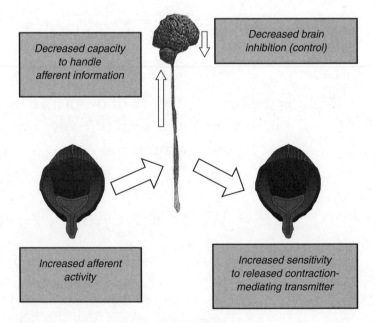

Figure 6 Pathophysiology of overactive bladder

OAB is defined as a combination of symptoms which include urgency with or without urge/urgency incontinence, often associated with frequency, and nocturia. The urgency is a sensation generally associated with a fear of leaking urine.

- Urgency is the complaint of a sudden compelling desire to void, which is difficult to defer.
- Urge or urgency incontinence is the complaint of involuntary loss of urine that is accompanied by or immediately preceded by urgency.
- Urinary frequency is the need to void more than eight times in a 24-hour period.
- Nocturia is the complaint that the individual has to wake at night one or more times to void.

10. What is urgency and how do I know I have it?

Urgency is defined as the complaint of a sudden compelling desire to void, which is difficult to defer. As one television advertisement for OAB described it, it is the feeling of "I gotta go." Urgency is not a normal sensation. For those with urine leakage associated with urgency (urgency incontinence) they may describe having little "warning time" between the onset of the sensation of urgency and the loss of control of urine. Most people with urgency feel that the sensation is strong enough that they need to stop what they are doing in order to get to the bathroom as quickly as possible to prevent urine leakage. Measurement of urgency is difficult and at present there is no widely agreed upon tool to measure the severity of urgency. Commonly urgency is measured by whether or not one can complete what one is doing when urgency occurs or whether one needs to abruptly stop what one is doing and rush to

Diagnosis of Overactive Bladder

the bathroom to prevent leakage. The most severe form of urgency is urgency incontinence.

Urgency is different than "urge to void." We all feel an urge to void. Typically, we may feel the urge to void when our bladder is one-third to one-half full. This signal alerts one to bladder filling. Should one choose to ignore or suppress this message and continue to hold one's urine, the sensation of urge will get progressively stronger until one is uncomfortable and chooses to urinate. This is a gradual buildup in the intensity, as opposed to urgency which is sudden, like the flip of a light switch.

11. Does everyone with OAB leak urine?

No, not everyone with OAB has urinary incontinence. In fact, two-thirds of individuals with OAB do not leak urine and are said to have "OAB dry." A larger percentage of men with OAB tend to be dry, whereas women more commonly experience urgency incontinence. There is variability in the severity of urinary incontinence. Some individuals may have urgency incontinence episodes only once or a few times per week, while others may wet three or more times per day. Remember, women also may have stress urinary incontinence (see Questions 5 to 7).

Individuals who do not leak urine may be just as bothered by their OAB symptoms as individuals who leak urine. Just because you don't leak urine doesn't mean that you don't deserve treatment. If your symptoms are bothersome, you should seek evaluation and treatment.

12. Are there medical conditions that may cause or mimic OAB?

There are a variety of conditions that may produce symptoms typical of OAB. Transient or reversible conditions include urinary tract infection, bladder stone(s), malignant or premalignant conditions of the bladder, drug side effects (see **Table 2**), excessive urine output, restricted mobility, severe constipation, and altered mental status (see **Table 3**). Other conditions that can contribute to, or may be associated with, OAB include obstruction to the outflow of urine from the bladder, **pelvic prolapse** (descent of the bladder and other pelvic organs out of the pelvis), and significant stress incontinence.

Potentially treatable causes of urinary incontinence which may be sudden or subacute in onset can be summarized by using the suggestive made up word DIAPPERS:

- Delirium—confusion
- Infection—urinary infection
- **Atrophic vaginitis**—low or absent estrogen levels before or after menopause or after hysterectomy and oophorectomy
- Pharmaceutical agents—medications
- Psychologic—depression, dementia
- Excess urine output—secondary to increased fluid intake, increased renal production of urine, or overflow incontinence
- Restricted mobility—difficulty with ambulation (walking) related to musculoskeletal problems or environmental factors
- Stool impaction—significant constipation

Pelvic prolapse

A weakening in the web of muscles at the base of the pelvis causing a protrusion of the bladder, urethra, uterus, or rectum into the vagina and possibly beyond (beyond the vaginal introitus).

Atrophic vaginitis

Changes in the vaginal lining and wall caused by low or absent estrogen levels before or after menopause or after hysterectomy and oophorectomy.

Table 2 Medications that may cause side effects that contribute to urinary incontinence

Alcohol	Increased urine volume, frequency, urgency, sedation, delirium
Alpha-agonists (e.g., pseudo-ephedrine, ephedrine)	Urinary retention
Alpha-blockers (e.g., tamsulosin [Flomax], doxazosin [Cardura], terazosin [Hytrin], alfuzosin [Uroxatral])	Urethral relaxation
ACE inhibitors, type I	Increased urine volume, cough with relaxation of pelvic floor
Anticholinergics (e.g., Darifenacin [Enablex], Fesoterodine [Toviaz], oxybutynin [Ditropan], Solifenacin [Vesicare], tolterodine [Detrol], Trospium chloride [Sanctura])	Urinary retention, overflow incontinence, stool impaction
Antidepressants (e.g., imipramine [Tofranil])	See anticholinergic side effects, sedation
Antiparkinsonism medications	Urinary urgency, constipation
Antipsychotics	See anticholinergic side effects, sedation, rigidity
Beta-agonists	Urinary retention
Caffeine	Bladder irritability that may aggravate or cause urge incontinence
Calcium-channel blockers	Urinary retention
Diuretics	Increased urine volume, urinary frequency, urgency
Sedatives/hypnotics	Sedation, delirium, immobility

Table 3   Management of conditions that cause reversible urinary incontinence

Condition	Management
Difficulty getting to or unwillingness to go to the toilet	
Delirium	Identification and management of the cause of the confused state of mind
Impaired mobility	Regular toileting, use of toilet substitutes (i.e., bedside commode, urinal)
Psychological problems	Appropriate psychological therapy
Drug side effects	If appropriate, discontinuation or decreased dosage of the drug, or changing to an alternative drug
Increased urine production	
Hyperglycemia	Improved control of blood sugars
Hypercalcemia	Treatment of the cause of the hypercalcemia
Excess fluid intake	Restriction of fluid intake and avoidance of caffeinated fluids
Fluid overload	**Diuretics**
Venous insufficiency with lower extremity edema	Support hose (TEDs), elevation of legs, low sodium diet
Congestive heart failure	Medical therapy to optimize cardiac function
Urinary tract infection	Antibiotic therapy
Atrophic vaginitis/ urethritis	Topical estrogen therapy if not at risk for use of estrogen therapy
Stool impaction	Disimpaction (manual removal of stool), institution of therapy to prevent constipation including: increased fiber and fluids, stool softeners, and/or laxatives if needed

Diagnosis of Overactive Bladder

13. What causes OAB?

The primary causes of OAB are not well defined. The mechanism for over activity of the bladder may be related to a problem with nerves, a neurogenic cause (i.e., something starting from or caused by the nerves themselves), or a problem with the bladder muscle itself, but there also may be other causes. The central nervous system, which includes the brain and the spinal cord, controls bladder function in a manner similar to an on-off circuit that you are able to voluntarily control. Damage to certain areas of the brain and spinal cord may alter this control and lead to bladder over activity. Neurological conditions that may be associated with OAB include stroke (cerebrovascular accident, CVA), Parkinson's disease, multiple sclerosis, and spinal cord injury. Conditions that may lead to alterations in the bladder muscle function include bladder outlet obstruction, such as in men with benign enlargement of the prostate gland (BPH), or aging. Specialized studies of bladder function, called urodynamic studies (discussed in Question 30), have demonstrated an age-related decrease in the capacity of the bladder, and an increased incidence of detrusor overactivity, a decreased force of the urine stream, and a decreased volume of urine voided along with incomplete bladder emptying. Changes in the muscarinic receptors in the bladder may also occur with aging. In a European study, some aspects of diet and lifestyle were associated with an increased risk of developing OAB. These factors included soda intake, being overweight or obese, and smoking.

Lastly, changes in the sensory (afferent) pathway, the nerves that carry the sensations of bladder filling to the brain, may contribute to OAB. Nerves within the bladder wall and lining (urothelium) respond to stretching of the bladder (such as during bladder filling and noxious stimuli) by sending messages (nerve impulses) to the brain via the spinal cord, and these messages tell the brain that the bladder needs to respond. The brain then sends impulses to the bladder (**efferent pathway**) to tell the bladder to contract. Thus, abnormalities in the **afferent pathway** may lead to the sensation of urgency and/or over activity in the efferent pathway, which is responsible for bladder contractions (**Figure 6**).

Conditions that can mimic OAB include:

- Urinary tract infections
- Bladder outlet obstruction
  - Males
    + Benign enlargement of the prostate
    + Cancerous (malignant) enlargement of the prostate
    + Urethral stricture (scarring of the urethra leading to narrowing)
    + Dysfunctional voiding (failing to relax the pelvic floor muscles with urination)
  - Females
    + Bladder outlet obstruction secondary to prior surgery for stress urinary incontinence
    + Dysfunctional voiding (see above)
- Decreased bladder contractility (incomplete bladder emptying may lead to urinary frequency)
- Bladder tumors or premalignant conditions may be associated with frequency and urgency and often hematuria, blood in the urine which may be visible (gross hematuria), or noticed just under the microscope (microscopic hematuria)

Efferent pathway

Messages (nerve impulse signals) outflowing from the central nervous system to the organs (the bladder for example).

Afferent pathway

Messages (nerve impulse signals) inflowing to the central nervous system (brain and spinal cord) from the bladder/urethra.

Diagnosis of Overactive Bladder

- Bladder stones may cause irritation of the bladder leading to frequency and urgency
- Interstitial cystitis/bladder pain syndrome
- Estrogen deficiency (inflammation from atrophic vaginitis can contribute to urgency)
- Stress urinary incontinence (in some women with stress incontinence, leakage of urine into the proximal urethra may lead to urgency)
- Neurologic causes
  - Cerebrovascular accident (stroke)
  - Multiple sclerosis
  - Dementia including Alzheimer's
  - Spinal cord injury
  - Diabetes
  - Parkinson's disease

14. How common is OAB?

OAB is a very common condition. Previous studies estimated that up to 17% of adult Americans suffer from OAB and that worldwide this affects between 50 and 100 million individuals. More recent studies suggest that the prevalence of OAB may be even greater. OAB affects both males and females. The prevalence of OAB increases with age for both males and females (see **Figure 7**).

Urgency incontinence is more frequently seen in women than in men. Thus, women have a greater chance of being "OAB wet," and men are more likely to be "OAB dry."

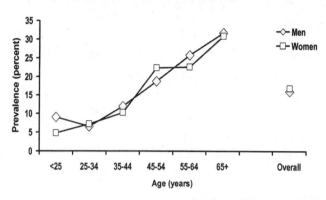

Figure 7   Prevalence of overactive bladder

Adapted from Stewart WF, van Rooten JB, Cundiff GW, Abrams P, Hezzog AR et al. Prevalence of Overactive Bladder in US. World J Urol 2002. Reprinted with permission from Springer-Verlag.

15. What is the natural history of OAB? Is it permanent? Can it resolve or does it come and go?

There is little information regarding the natural history (course over time) of OAB. The few studies that are available suggest that OAB is a chronic condition in adults that persists symptomatically. There may be exacerbations and improvements in symptoms depending on lifestyle, dietary changes, and variation in stress and other factors which we do not understand. The good news is that the symptoms often can be controlled with a combination of behavioral modification and medication.

16. I had problems with urinary frequency and controlling my urine as a child. Did I have OAB then?

Children can develop OAB. In fact, OAB is one of the most common causes of lower urinary tract dysfunction in children. It is thought that OAB in children is a transient condition that resolves with time, but two recent studies have demonstrated that adult women with OAB symptoms and urinary incontinence have a higher incidence of childhood lower urinary tract symptoms. Thus, childhood symptoms may predict adult symptoms. Further long-term studies will be needed to determine whether or not OAB symptoms in children persist or progress into adulthood.

17. When are people at risk for developing OAB?

OAB affects children and adults. The prevalence increases with age. More recent studies assessing the prevalence of OAB have demonstrated that OAB symptoms occur in adults as early as the 40s with a greater percentage of older adults being affected. The prevalence of OAB symptoms increases with age in both males and females (see Figure 7, Question 14). In males, OAB symptoms may develop in combination with bladder outlet obstruction related to enlargement of the prostate.

18. Is OAB hereditary?

There is little information available regarding the genetics of OAB. In studies of twins, there was a suggestion that OAB with urgency incontinence may be hereditary in some cases. In children with OAB there is often a family member with OAB. In a recent study of female urinary incontinence, hereditary factors did appear to play a role in the development of urinary incontinence in women. The study found that there was an increased risk for any type of incontinence, that is, stress or mixed (stress plus urgency), and severe symptoms for women whose mothers or older sisters were incontinent.

19. What is the impact of OAB?

OAB has a negative effect on quality of life. It is often associated with additional medical comorbidities and has a huge economic impact.

Studies evaluating the effect of OAB and urgency incontinence on quality of life have demonstrated that urgency incontinence has a greater negative effect on quality of life than stress incontinence. This is understandable when one considers that with stress incontinence the individual has an element of control. If he or she avoids coughing, laughing, sneezing, or exertion, then leaking can be avoided. With urgency incontinence, however, there is little to no warning or control.

When compared to several other disease states, individuals with urgency incontinence believed that they had a worse quality of life in several quality-of-life parameters than individuals who had diabetes mellitus. Only depressed patients rated their quality of life worse than individuals with urgency incontinence.

OAB and urinary incontinence may affect one's quality of life in a variety of ways:

- Psychological: may lead to guilt or depression, loss of self-esteem, fear of being a burden, and fear of lack of bladder control or the smell of urine odor.
- Social: may lead to a reduction in social interactions and limit travel to planning around toilet accessibility.
- Domestic: there is a need for specialized pads and protective underwear; if the individual is elderly, he or she may have to depend on a caregiver to obtain these items.
- Occupational: may lead to absences from work, decreased productivity, and difficulties with colleagues at work.
- Sexual: may lead to avoidance of sexual activity and intimacy.
- Physical: may lead to limitation or cessation of physical activity, particularly in those individuals who suffer from mixed incontinence.

Studies have demonstrated that urinary incontinence is the reason for nursing home admission in about 50% of nursing home patients. In the elderly, urinary incontinence is associated with an increased risk of urinary tract infections, skin infections, and irritation. Furthermore, there is an association between OAB and urinary incontinence and risk of falls and bone fractures in older women. The increased risk of falls may well be due to having to rush to the bathroom.

Individuals with nocturia may note lack of energy, chronic fatigue, or difficulty performing daily activities. Nocturia itself affects quality of life, leads to disturbed sleep, and has a negative effect on overall health.

The overall economic burden of urge incontinence is extremely high. In 1995, it was estimated to be 17.5 billion dollars, which exceeded the economic burden for breast cancer or pneumonia. This economic burden reflects the inclusion of costs of pads and diapers, laundry costs, treatment for urinary tract infections, skin infections/irritation, and medical therapy for OAB. In addition, there are additional costs that are difficult to measure, such as the time spent by a caregiver and nursing home care related to urinary incontinence.

20. Is OAB treatable?

Yes, OAB is treatable. Most individuals will note a significant improvement in their symptoms with a combination of behavioral modification and medical therapy (see Questions 32 to 56). Although each of these therapies is effective alone, the best results are noted when they are used in combination. Those individuals who do not improve with medical therapy and behavioral modification, or for whom medical therapy is contraindicated (i.e., medically inappropriate), may be treated with other forms of therapy, including sacral neuromodulation (see Questions 71 to 75). Investigational therapies for the treatment of OAB include intravesical instillations of resiniferatoxin (RTX) and injection of botulinum toxin into the bladder wall (see Questions 63 to 67). Rarely, the OAB symptoms may be refractory to all these therapies (i.e., the therapy doesn't work). Then bladder augmentation procedures, procedures to enlarge the bladder, may be considered (see Questions 77 to 80).

Management of OAB

* First line therapies for OAB
  + Behavioral therapy
  + Medical therapy

- Second line therapies for OAB
  + Sacral neuromodulation
- Third line therapies for OAB (currently investigational and not approved by the FDA)
  + Injection of botulinum toxin
  + Intravesical instillation of resiniferatoxin
- Last resort therapies for OAB
  + Bladder augmentation
  + Bladder denervation procedures

When you discuss therapy for OAB, it is important that you and your healthcare provider discuss the expectations of the treatment. For example, if you are currently voiding 20 times per day and have 5 incontinent episodes per day, a reasonable expectation may be a reduction in your urinary frequency by 20 percent and your incontinence episodes by 70%. If you expect to be dry all the time and void only six times per day with therapy, this expectation may not be realistic.

21. I think I have OAB. Do I see my regular general practitioner or should I see a specialist?

If you think you have OAB symptoms it is important that you discuss this first with your primary care provider. A lot of primary care providers feel comfortable evaluating and treating OAB, and if they don't they will refer you to either a **urologist** or a **urogynecologist**. Studies have shown that patients tend to cope with their symptoms for several years before discussing them with their healthcare provider. Unfortunately, studies have also shown that healthcare providers often don't screen for OAB and, even if a diagnosis is made, don't always treat patients for OAB. So, if you

Urologist

A specialist in the area of the male and female urinary tact, male genitalia and male and female pelvis.

Urogynecologist

A specialist with advanced training and practice in the fields of gynecology as well as the study, diagnosis and treatment of the female genitourinary tract.

bring up your concerns regarding your bladder symptoms and your healthcare provider doesn't appear concerned and doesn't discuss how he/she is going to evaluate and treat your symptoms, don't lose hope; seek out a urologist or urogynecologist. If you don't know of a specific individual in your community, you can get assistance in identifying the healthcare provider with an interest in treating bladder troubles by talking to the receptionist in the local urology or urogynecology practice(s). Many healthcare providers will identify their specialty interests to make it easier for patients to select the correct healthcare provider. Similarly, if you are being treated by your primary care provider and you are not seeing any change in your symptoms, you should consider seeing a specialist.

Other indications to see a specialist are:

- If you have had blood in your urine
- If you have a history of recurrent urinary tract infections
- If you have had prior pelvic surgery
- If you have had prior surgery for stress urinary incontinence
- If you have pelvic organ prolapse (**cystocele:** when the bladder drops down into the vagina; **rectocele:** when the rectum bulges into the vagina; **enterocele:** the intestine bulging into the vagina)
- If you have pelvic pain and/or pain with urination
- If you are not emptying your bladder well

22. Is OAB curable?

Medical therapy in combination with behavioral modification improves OAB symptoms in up to 75% of individuals. This does not mean that all of these individuals

Cystocele

Hernia-like disorder in women that occurs when the wall between the bladder and the vagina weakens and the bladder drops into the vagina.

Rectocele

Occurs when the fascia—a wall of fibrous tissue separating the rectum from the vagina— becomes weakened, allowing the front wall of the rectum to bulge into the vagina.

Enterocele

Occurs when your small intestine (small bowel) drops into the lower pelvic cavity and protrudes into your vagina, creating a bulge. An enterocele is a vaginal hernia.

are dry and that none of them continue to experience urgency and frequency. Medical therapy rarely "cures" people, meaning total lack of symptoms. However, the initial goal of medical therapy is to achieve a significant improvement in quality of life while the patient is taught and helped to control the condition with a combination of behavioral changes, improvement in pelvic muscle control, and medications.

23. Can men have prostate problems and OAB or is it all just related to the prostate?

Lower urinary tract
symptoms (LUTS)

Term used to describe storage and emptying symptoms.

Lower urinary tract symptoms (LUTS) is a term used to describe two types of lower urinary tract symptoms: emptying and storage symptoms. Men with enlarged prostates will often present with emptying symptoms, such as a slow stream, hesitancy, intermittent stream, and straining; they may also experience post-void dribbling. These symptoms are often related to the obstruction of urine outflow from the enlarged prostate. Approximately 40% to 60% of men with prostatic enlargement and bladder outlet obstruction also have storage symptoms including daytime frequency, nocturia, urgency, and, less commonly, urgency incontinence. These irritative symptoms are suggestive of an OAB. The fact that up to 30 to 35% of men with benign enlargement of the prostate who undergo surgical treatment for their prostatic enlargement still suffer from storage symptoms after the treatment suggests that they truly have two conditions: obstruction due to the prostatic enlargement and OAB. In many individuals, however, successful treatment of the prostatic obstruction will improve the OAB symptoms. Why this occurs is not fully understood.

Because it appears that men with prostatic enlargement can suffer from symptoms related to the obstruction and may also have OAB, current studies are underway that are looking at the use of medical therapy to simultaneously treat both of these symptoms. Limited studies have demonstrated that it is feasible to use a combination of medications used for prostatic enlargement, such as alpha blockers and anticholinergics. Examples of such alpha blockers include: alfuzosin (Uroxatral), doxazosin (Cardura), silodosin (Rapaflo) tamsulosin (Flomax), and terazosin (Hytrin). Examples of the oral anticholinergics include: darifenacin (Enablex), fesoterodine (Toviaz), oxybutynin patch (Oxytrol) (Ditropan and Ditropan XL), oxybutynin patch (Oxytrol), oxybutynin gel (Gelnique), solifenacin (Vesicare), tolterodine (Detrol IR and Detrol LA), and tropsium chloride (Sanctura and Sanctura XR).

24. Is waking up at night caused by OAB?

Nocturia is defined as the complaint that an individual has to wake at night one or more times to void. Nocturia is very common, and it appears that the incidence and severity increases as one gets older. Most people over 65 years of age get up at least one time at night to urinate. In one European study, 10% of the general population age 20 years and older suffered from nocturia two or more times per night. In addition, this study demonstrated that nocturia has a significant impact on one's quality of life and that there was a correlation between the number of times one awakened at night to void and the impact on quality of life. Nocturia is often present with OAB, but there are several other conditions that can cause nocturia, including:

- Cardiovascular disease, including congestive heart failure and circulatory problems
- Diabetes mellitus
- Diabetes insipidus, which is a condition that is either related to a brain or kidney problem and results in the overproduction of urine
- Sleep apnea, which is a breathing problem that occurs during sleep
- Lower urinary tract obstruction such as that related to prostate enlargement
- Primary sleep disorders
- Behavioral and environmental factors
- Nocturnal polyuria, whereby the urine output over the course of the entire day is normal, but the urine output at night is in excess of what is normal
- Polyuria, whereby the total urine output for the entire day is excessive

Frequency volume chart

A document plotting the amount of urine and number of times an individual urinates over a period of time.

To determine whether the nocturia is related to OAB requires that your healthcare provider review your history, medications, and a **frequency volume chart**. A frequency volume chart or bladder diary allows your healthcare provider to determine the potential cause of your nocturia (see Question 38). Treatment of the nocturia will vary with the cause. Preliminary studies have demonstrated, however, that if some of the episodes of nocturia are due to OAB, the use of antimuscarinics will help to decrease these OAB voids at night, but only these.

25. Why does the number of times I get up at night seem out of proportion (greater) with the number of times I urinate during the day? What can I do about this?

It is puzzling that you can be awake for say 16 hours during the day and be asleep for only 8 hours and actually urinate on a more frequent hourly basis during the 8 hours that you are "sleeping" than during the 16 hours that you are awake. There are several factors that can cause this.

During the daytime, during periods of inactivity when you are sitting or standing in one position for long periods there is pooling of blood in your legs, "venous stasis." This leads to a leakage of fluid through the vessel walls into the tissues called edema. At night, this fluid is resorbed back into the blood stream. The kidneys compensate for this increase in volume by making more urine.

Another cause of awakening at night to urinate is a decrease in the release of a chemical, vasopressin, at night. Vasopressin is a chemical that is released by a part of the brain. Vasopressin stimulates the kidneys to hold onto fluid and to make less urine. So, for example, on a hot, humid day when one is sweating a lot, the brain releases more vasopressin to tell the kidneys to make less urine and hold onto fluid so that dehydration does not occur. In some people, the amount of vasopressin that is produced at night decreases as they get older.

Some individuals take diuretics more than once a day. Taking a diuretic late in the afternoon or at night may increase the amount of urine produced at night and the frequency of urination at night.

Sleep disorders, including sleep apnea, can cause nocturia. Sleep apnea is a condition whereby during sleep the soft structures in the throat relax and close off the airway. Waking occurs to reopen the airway. Symptoms of sleep apnea include: snoring, restless sleep with frequent awakenings, daytime sleepiness, and morning headaches. Obesity may be associated with sleep apnea.

Congestive heart failure, a problem with the pumping ability of the heart, can cause peripheral pooling of blood and "leakage" of serum into the tissues outside of the blood vessels (edema). At night with less stress on the heart, and with changes in position, the fluid is resorbed back into the blood stream.

Too much fluid intake at night, particularly if one drinks caffeine (coffee, tea, soda) or alcohol-containing fluids at night.

Decreased nocturnal bladder capacity means that the bladder holds less urine at night than it does in the daytime.

Diabetes mellitus may result in nocturia if one's blood sugars are elevated at night and more urine production results.

Diabetes insipidus, a disorder in which there is either not enough vasopressin produced or the kidneys don't respond to vasopressin, can increase urine output during the day and night.

26. What can someone do about nocturia?

Your healthcare provider may ask you to make note of how many times you void during the day and night, to measure the amount of urine that you void during the day and the night, and to keep track of the volume, type, and time of fluid intake throughout the day and night. This information along with the other parts of your history and physical examination and **urinalysis** may help your healthcare provider identify the cause of your nocturia and the best treatment.

There are simple things that you can try to improve your nocturia. Restrict your fluid intake in the late afternoon and evening, cut out caffeinated and alcohol-based drinks in the evening, elevate your legs during the day or consider support/compression stockings if you have problems with swelling of your legs.

If you take diuretics (water pills such as furosemide [Lasix], hydrochlorothiazide [HydroDiuril, Microzide]) at night, taking them earlier in the day may help improve your nocturia (overall urinary frequency may remain the same but the timing may change).

If you have associated daytime OAB symptoms, then you may notice an improvement in your nocturia with the use of OAB medications.

If your healthcare provider feels that you are making too much urine at night, despite restricting your fluid intake, and your bladder size is normal, your healthcare provider may recommend a medication called Desmopressin (DDAVP). Desmopressin is a synthetic (man-made) chemical that mimics vasopressin. Thus, when

Urinalysis
A type of test of the urine to determine normalcy or abnormality.

taken at night, it causes the kidneys to make less urine at night. It only lasts in your system for about 8 hours and thus the following day your body gets rid of the fluid that you held onto at night. Side effects of desmopressin include dry mouth, mood changes, and sleep disturbances. **Rarely, desmopressin can lower the salt (sodium) level in the body and if the sodium level is lowered too quickly or too much it can cause a seizure**. Therefore, individuals taking desmopressin must refrain from drinking fluids in the evening, and periodic blood tests are needed to monitor salt (sodium) levels in the blood.

27. How is OAB diagnosed?

OAB is a condition with symptoms that are suggestive of detrusor overactivity, in the setting of no identifiable metabolic or pathologic conditions that mimic or cause OAB. The evaluation has two purposes: (1) to determine whether the individual's symptoms are suggestive of OAB, and (2) to rule out those metabolic or pathologic conditions that may cause or mimic OAB. The initial evaluation starts with an analysis of your symptoms to determine whether they are consistent with OAB. Remember, those individuals with OAB suffer from urgency with or without urgency incontinence and will often have frequency and nocturia (see Question 9). Simplified bladder health questionnaires allow the healthcare provider to screen for possible bladder troubles. The following questions are often asked.

Over the past four weeks:

- Did you wake up at night to urinate two or more times?

- Did you have a sudden and uncomfortable feeling that you had to urinate soon?
- Were you bothered or concerned about bladder control?
- Did you lose or leak urine for any reason?
- Did you wear a pad or other material to absorb urine that you may have lost?

Symptom Assessment

A symptom assessment will focus on your urinary symptoms, ask how often you urinate, whether you have urgency, and if there is leakage. The healthcare provider will ask whether straining, coughing, laughing, or sneezing induces leakage. It is often helpful for you to complete a voiding diary over several days to better clarify your urinary symptoms (see **Figure 8**). In addition, your healthcare provider will want to know how bothered you are by these symptoms. If you are not bothered, then unless you are suffering from recurrent

Diagnosis of Overactive Bladder

Optional Tools for Consideration:
Voiding Log/Bladder Diary

Day 1   Date: __/__/__   Number of pads used today: _____

TIME	FLUIDS		URINATION					ACCIDENTS		
	What did you drink?	How much?	How many times?	How much each time? (S = small, M = moderate, L = large)	Did you have to rush to the bathroom?	Did you hurt yourself or fall down rushing to the bathroom?	What activity did it interrupt?	Did you have any accidents this time? (Sudden loss of urine)	How much urine did you leak? (S = small, M = moderate, L = large)	What were you doing at the time? (Exercising, sleeping, relaxing, etc.)
SAMPLE 12 PM	Juice	Tall glass	1	(S) M L	(Yes) No	Yes (No)	Walking the dog	(Yes) No	(S) M L	Gardening
				S M L	Yes No	Yes No		Yes No	S M L	
				S M L	Yes No	Yes No		Yes No	S M L	
				S M L	Yes No	Yes No		Yes No	S M L	
				S M L	Yes No	Yes No		Yes No	S M L	
				S M L	Yes No	Yes No		Yes No	S M L	
				S M L	Yes No	Yes No		Yes No	S M L	
				S M L	Yes No	Yes No		Yes No	S M L	
				S M L	Yes No	Yes No		Yes No	S M L	
				S M L	Yes No	Yes No		Yes No	S M L	

Notes: _____   13

Figure 8 Sample of a voiding diary

urinary tract or skin infections, there is no need to treat you. During the symptom assessment, the healthcare provider will try to determine whether your symptoms are suggestive of OAB, stress incontinence, or a combination of the two. As part of your symptom assessment, your healthcare provider may ask you to complete a voiding diary for 3 to 5 days to better understand your fluid intake and symptoms (see Figure 8).

History and Physical Examination

A medical history, physical examination, and a urinalysis are helpful in ruling out other conditions that mimic or cause OAB (see Question 12). During the history component, your healthcare provider will want to know about your prior and current medical and surgical histories, what medications you are taking, and if you have allergies. Questions about the medical status of your relatives may be asked. In addition, several questions pertaining to dietary and lifestyle issues will be asked. These may include: how much fluid you typically drink during the day, how much caffeinated fluid you drink, your occupation, and your ease of access to restrooms at work. The physical examination will focus on your lower abdomen and perineum. Often a brief neurological evaluation will be included. The healthcare provider will palpate your lower abdomen to see if your bladder is distended. In women, a pelvic examination is performed to determine if there is significant pelvic prolapse. During the examination of the perineum in women, the healthcare provider may ask you to strain/bear down or cough to determine if there is any loss of control of urine. Some healthcare providers may put a small Q-tip into the urethra and then ask you to strain to see if there is a significant deflection of the Q-tip suggestive of stress urinary incontinence. A rectal examination is often performed to check anal muscle tone. In males, the rectal examination includes a prostate examination, to check the size of the prostate, and to determine if there are nodules that may indicate the presence of prostate cancer.

Urinalysis

A urinalysis is a helpful test to rule out a urinary tract infection. In addition, the presence of red blood cells in the urine in the absence of a urinary tract infection would require further evaluation to rule out a bladder tumor or stone as the cause of the blood cells in the urine and the voiding symptoms needs to be ruled out. The presence of an excessive amount of glucose in the urine would prompt further evaluation for diabetes, and the presence of an excessive amount of protein in the urine would prompt further evaluation for kidney diseases. A very dilute urine is suggestive of either drinking excessive amounts of fluid or an inability of the kidney to hold fluids back.

Additional Studies

Depending on your age, voiding symptoms, and prior medical and surgical history, you may need additional studies. In men with symptoms suggestive of obstruction from an enlarged prostate, elderly patients, patients with recurrent urinary tract infections, and those with neurological diseases, the healthcare provider may perform an **ultrasound** scan of the bladder after urination to ensure that the bladder is emptying properly. The machine will calculate an estimated volume of urine in the bladder. Less commonly, a catheter may be passed through the urethra into the bladder to drain the bladder and measure the **post-void residual urine** volume.

Ultrasound

A noninvasive test using radio waves (frequency greater than 30,000 MHz); used to evaluate the kidneys and bladder to assess bladder emptying capacity.

Post-void residual urine

The amount of urine left in the bladder after voiding; if elevated may lead to urinary tract infections, bladder stones, further distention of the bladder, worsening of bladder function, or dilation of the kidneys and ureter.

Younger individuals should be able to empty their bladder to completion. As one gets older, there is an anticipated small amount of urine that may be left behind after urinating. Post-void residuals greater than 100 cc to 150 cc are considered to be very abnormal and suggestive of either outlet obstruction or poor bladder function. Rarely will any additional studies be needed to initially begin treatment. Those individuals with red blood cells in the urine will need to undergo a cystoscopy and an X-ray of their kidneys and ureters. Cystoscopy is a procedure in which the bladder and urethra are examined through a narrow telescope-like device that is passed through the urethra into the bladder. In those individuals with complex medical problems, prior bladder or urethral surgery, and those who have failed prior therapies for OAB, a urodynamic study may be indicated (see Question 30).

28. What happens if my urinalysis shows red blood cells in it? Do I need additional tests?

The presence of red blood cells in the urine is called hematuria. Hematuria may be gross, meaning that the blood is visible, or microscopic, meaning it is visible only with an examination through a microscope and the urine is not red or pink. Both microscopic and gross hematuria require further evaluation. Typically the evaluation of hematuria includes X-ray tests to evaluate the kidneys and ureters (the tubes that drain the urine from the kidneys into the bladder) and the cystoscopy to evaluate the bladder and the urethra. In adults, the cystoscopy is often performed in the healthcare provider's office. A numbing gel is placed into the ure-thra first and then a small flexible telescope-like device, the cystoscope, is inserted through the urethra into the bladder. Fluid is run through the cystoscope to open the urethra and fill the bladder to make sure that the entire bladder and urethra are examined.

This evaluation is performed to rule out stones and tumors in the kidney, ureters, bladder, and urethra. It also rules out strictures (scars causing obstruction) in the ureters and urethra.

If red blood cells are noted in the urine, the urine sam-ple is also sent for cytology, specialized urine test by which the urine sample is examined for the presence of cancer cells.

If there are other abnormalities noted in your urine sam-ple or history and physical, your healthcare provider may recommend that you see a medical kidney specialist, a nephrologist, for further evaluation of the hematuria.

29. Are there screening tools that one can use to detect OAB?

At present there is no universally agreed upon screening tool. Efforts have been made to develop one that is reli-able and readily identifies those individuals with OAB.

The OAB V-8 is a simplified eight-question screening tool that has been shown to help identify individuals with OAB (see **Figure 9**).

The questions below ask about how bothered you may be by some bladder symptoms. Some people are bothered by bladder symptoms and may not realize that there are treatments available for their symptoms. *Please circle that number* that best describes how much you have been bothered by each symptom. Add the numbers together for a total score and record the score in the box provided at the bottom.

How bothered have you been by...	Not at all	A little bit	Some- what	Quite a bit	A great deal	A very great deal
1. Frequent urination during the daytime hours?	0	1	2	3	4	5
2. An uncomfortable urge to urinate?	0	1	2	3	4	5
3. A sudden urge to urinate with little or no warning?	0	1	2	3	4	5
4. Accidental loss of small amounts of urine?	0	1	2	3	4	5
5. Nighttime urination?	0	1	2	3	4	5
6. Waking up at night because you had to urinate?	0	1	2	3	4	5
7. An uncontrollable urge to urinate?	0	1	2	3	4	5
8. Urine loss associated with a strong desire to urinate?	0	1	2	3	4	5

Are you a male?   If male, ☐ add 2 points to your score.

Please add up your responses to the questions above ☐☐

Please hand this page to your doctor when you see him/her for your visit.

> **If your score is 8 or greater, you may have overactive bladder. There are effective treatments for this condition. You may want to talk with a healthcare professional about your symptoms.**

Figure 9 OAB Awareness Tool

30. What is a urodynamic study?

A urodynamic study is a test used to assess how well the bladder and urethra are performing their job of storing and releasing urine.

Urodynamic tests can help your healthcare provider assess such symptoms as the following:

- Urinary incontinence
- Urinary frequency
- Urgency
- Problems with starting one's stream (hesitancy)
- Painful urination
- Incomplete bladder emptying
- Infections

A urodynamic study is composed of a series of tests. Depending on your symptoms, you may need some or all of the components. Urodynamic studies are often performed in the healthcare provider's office or may be performed in a specialized outpatient area.

Little preparation is needed for a urodynamic test. You can eat prior to the test. Your healthcare provider may ask you to come in with a full bladder.

The urodynamic study may start with a uroflow. A **uroflow** is a noninvasive test in which you are asked to urinate into a specialized urine collection device that is able to measure how fast the urine exits your body. The uroflow measures the rate of urination in cubic centimeters or milliliters per second. After voiding, a specialized catheter is placed into your urethra and passed into your bladder. The catheter is taped in place to prevent it from falling out during the study. Your bladder is emptied and the volume left behind in your bladder after voiding, the Post-void Residual (PVR), is recorded. Once the catheter is secured in place and your bladder is emptied, the catheter is connected to a special pressure monitor, a transducer, and to the tubing that supplies the sterile fluid. A separate catheter is placed into your rectum, also connected to a transducer, which allows the healthcare provider to measure pressures within your abdomen. In order to assess the

Uroflow

The rate of flow of the urine stream; often a component of a urodynamic study, but may be performed in the office.

activity of your pelvic floor muscles skin patch electrodes or small needle electrodes will be placed in the area near your anus. These electrodes measure activity in your pelvic floor muscles, which also surround the urethra. This type of study is called **electromyography (EMG)**. The EMG measures activity in the muscles of the pelvic floor. During the urodynamic study, **fluoroscopy** (X-ray) may be used to visualize your bladder and urethra during bladder filling and voiding. If X-ray is used during the study it is called **video-urodynamics**.

After placement of the two catheters and the electrodes, the filling/storage phase of the urodynamic study, the **cystometrogram (CMG)** is started. Sterile fluid is instilled into your bladder at a rate specified by your healthcare provider. A computer screen displays the pressures in your abdomen and your bladder, and the activity of your pelvic floor muscles.

Shortly after starting the study you will be asked to cough or bear down. This is to ensure that the catheters are in the correct position and the pressure sensors (transducers) are working properly. While your bladder is filling with the sterile fluid, your healthcare provider will ask you to indicate when you first feel the urge to void and when you feel a strong urge to void. The volumes in your bladder at each of these times will be recorded. If you have incontinence, your healthcare provider will ask you to bear down or cough periodically throughout the study to see if there is any urine leakage indicative of stress urinary incontinence. If urine leakage occurs, the bladder pressure at which it occurred is also recorded.

Electromyography (EMG)

Recording of the electric potentials from your pelvic floor muscles (spincter muscles) during bladder filling and emptying.

Fluoroscopy

Visualization of tissues and deep structures of the body by X-ray.

Video-urodynamics

Use of intermittent fluoroscopy (taking X-rays) during the urodynamic study to visualize the bladder and urethra.

Cystometrogram (CMG)

Recording of bladder pressure during filling and emptying.

Normally during bladder filling the bladder pressure remains very low and stable until one feels the urge to urinate and decides to void. During voiding, the bladder pressure quickly increases and then promptly decreases as soon as urination is completed. Periodic involuntary increases in bladder pressure during the study are referred to as detrusor overactivity (DO) and may contribute to the symptoms of frequency, urgency, and urgency incontinence. The CMG also evaluates bladder compliance. Bladder compliance is the ability of the bladder to hold increasing amounts of urine without increases in bladder pressure and reflects the elasticity of the bladder. Poor compliance, the inability to store urine at low pressures, may cause damage to the kidneys and be a source of urine leakage.

During the study, when you feel a strong urge to urinate, the fluid infusion will be stopped and you will be asked to void. During urination the bladder pressures and the urine flow rate are monitored. These values are then plotted on a nomogram called a pressure flow study. This study is particularly helpful in males as it helps determine if there is any significant obstruction to the outflow of urine. During voiding, the flow rate and electromyogram (EMG) are assessed. This is helpful in ensuring that there is appropriate relaxation of the pelvic floor muscles prior to voiding and that this relaxation continues throughout voiding.

In some cases, a specialized dye is used to fill your bladder. This allows your healthcare provider to take X-rays periodically during the study to look at your bladder and urethra. This final addition makes the study a "video-urodynamic" study.

31. Should every patient with OAB undergo urodynamics?

Not every patient with OAB symptoms needs to have urodynamic studies performed. Often patients with OAB symptoms are initially started on behavioral and medical therapy, either alone or in combination. If an individual fails to improve with these therapies, a urodynamic study may be performed prior to trying second line therapies such as neuromodulation or investigational therapies such as botulinum toxin.

If you experience urinary incontinence and your healthcare provider is concerned about whether or not there is stress incontinence, a urodynamic study may help identify the cause of your incontinence. Similarly, if you have had prior pelvic surgery for urinary incontinence and have persistent or a new onset of OAB symptoms after your surgery, your healthcare provider may want to perform a urodynamic study to ensure that there is no obstruction to the outflow of urine.

In men with lower urinary tract symptoms, a urodynamic study can be helpful in determining whether or not the symptoms are related to obstruction from the prostate, an OAB, or a combination of the two.

PART THREE

Treatment of Overactive Bladder

What are the options for treating OAB?

What are pelvic floor muscle exercises (Kegel exercises)?

What is neuromodulation/sacral nerve stimulation?

What is bladder augmentation?

More . . .

Behaviorial therapy

A group of treatments designed for educating an individual about his/her medical condition and the function of the organ affected so strategies can be developed to minimize or eliminate the symptoms.

32. What are the treatment options for OAB?

There are a variety of treatment options available for the management of OAB. These options vary from less invasive therapies, such as **behavioral therapy** and oral drug therapies, to more invasive therapies, such as instillation of compounds into the bladder, electrical stimulation, injection into the bladder wall, and surgical treatments. Typically you begin with the less invasive therapies first, reserving the intravesical and surgical therapies for those who fail behavioral and oral therapies.

First-line therapies for the management of OAB include:

- Behavioral therapy (see **Figure 10**)
- Pharmacologic therapy—anti-muscarinic medications

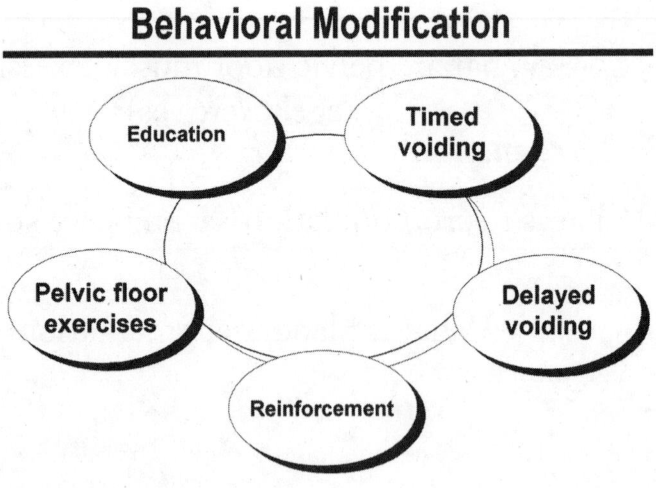

Behavioral Modification

Figure 10   Behavioral therapy
Types of behavioral therapy and management of symptoms.

Medications approved in the United States:

- Darifenacin
- Fesoterodine
- Oxybutynin (oxybutynin, Oxybutynin XL)
- Solifenacin
- Tolterodine (Tolterodine IR and ER)
- Transdermal Oxybutynin Gel and patch
- Trospium chloride (BID and XL)

Medications approved only in Europe

- Propiverine

Second-line therapies include:

- Sacral neuromodulation—electrical stimulation
- Injection of botulinum toxin into the bladder wall (investigational)
- Intravesical therapy—capsaicin and **resiniferatoxin** (investigational)

Third-line therapies (desperate measures) include:

- **Bladder augmentation**
- Urinary diversion (a desperate measure)

33. Are men and women with OAB symptoms treated the same?

Men may be treated differently than women. This is because many men with OAB symptoms often have symptoms related to bladder outlet obstruction from benign prostatic enlargement.

Urinary symptoms in men and women are referred to as lower urinary tract symptoms (LUTS). LUTS may be divided into filling/storage and voiding/emptying symptoms.

Resiniferatoxin

A chemical derived from a cactus-like plant, Euphorbia resinifera, which may be instilled into the bladder to decrease bladder activity.

Bladder augmentation

A surgical procedure whereby the bladder is enlarged with patches of organ tissue from the colon.

53

- Storage/filling symptoms include frequency, urgency, nocturia, and urgency incontinence.
- Emptying/voiding symptoms include poor urine stream, hesitancy, terminal dribbling, and feeling of incomplete emptying.

In males with LUTS, voiding symptoms are more common, but the filling/storage (OAB) symptoms are more bothersome.

Because many men present with both OAB and voiding symptoms, and because of the risk of urinary retention in men with benign prostatic enlargement, most men with LUTS are initially treated for prostatic enlargement and the voiding symptoms. If after treating the voiding symptoms, OAB symptoms persist and the male is emptying his bladder adequately, then treatment of the OAB with medical therapy is started.

Medications that are used to treat the voiding symptoms in men presumed to be due to obstruction by an enlarged prostate include alpha-adrenergic receptor blockers and 5-alpha-reductase inhibitors.

- Alpha-adrenergic receptor blockers are medications used to relax the muscle fibers in the prostate and bladder neck to relieve pressure and allow urine to flow more freely through the urethra. There are several different alpha-blockers available. Side effects of alpha-blockers may include dizziness when changing positions (postural hypotension), fatigue and headache, and ejaculatory dysfunction (less or no semen out the urethra with orgasm). It is recommended that alpha-blockers be taken in the evening just before going to bed to minimize the risk of dizziness.

- Alfuzosin (uroxatral): Alfuzosin does not require dose adjustment (titration) and is available as a single 10mg oral dose once a day. Ejaculatory dysfunction (decreased semen volume or anejaculation) is less common with alfuzosin.
- Doxazosin (cardura): Doxazosin is a titratable form of alpha-blocker that also may be associated with dizziness. Dose titration is recommended as well as taking the medication in the evening before going to bed. The dose ranges from 2mg to 8mg per day.
- Silodosin (Rapaflo): A new alpha-adrenergic receptor blocker available as a single 8mg dose therapy. May cause retrograde ejaculation.
- Tamsulosin (Flomax): Tamsulosin may decrease semen (ejaculate) volume or eliminate it entirely. Tamsulosin does not require titration. The recommended oral dose is 0.4mg daily, taken $\frac{1}{2}$ hour following the same meal each day.
- Terazosin (hytrin): Terazosin is a titratable form of alpha-blocker with doses ranging from 2mg to 10mg per day. Dose titration is recommended as well as taking the medication in the evening before going to bed.

- 5 alpha-reductase inhibitors are medications that interfere with the effect of certain male hormones (testosterone) on the prostate. By decreasing the levels in the prostate, these medications slow the growth of the prostate and subsequently cause it to decrease in size. It may take 6 to 12 months for these medications to exert their maximal effect. They also decrease the PSA (prostate specific antigen) by approximately 50%. Side effects of these medications may include decreased sex drive (libido), troubles with ejaculation, erectile troubles, and rarely breast tenderness and enlargement. In one study the problems with decreased sex drive and erectile troubles resolved after 1 year of use. The 5 alpha-reductase inhibitors work best in men with large prostates. There are two 5 alpha-reductase inhibitors available: finasteride (proscar) and dutasteride (avodart).

34. What is behavioral therapy?

The term behavioral therapy or behavioral modification encompasses a group of treatment methods that presume that an individual can be educated about his/her medical condition and can develop strategies to minimize or eliminate the symptoms (see Figure 10, in Question 32). For those individuals with OAB, the goals of behavioral therapy are to reduce or eliminate the number of incontinence episodes, the urgency episodes, and the urinary frequency. In individuals with urgency incontinence, there is a problem with the bladder and the **pelvic floor muscles**. Thus, behavioral therapy focuses on both the bladder and the pelvic floor muscles. There are several components to behavioral therapy (see Figure 10, Question 32). Behavioral therapy starts with patient education. The patient must understand normal lower urinary tract anatomy and function and the role of intelligent fluid restriction. Furthermore, the role of the bladder and the pelvic floor muscles in voiding and maintenance of continence must be understood. Patients are taught the role of **timed or prophylactic voiding** and how to use rapid pelvic floor contractions (quick flicks) to abort the sensation of urgency. Timed voiding is the process whereby one voids at regular intervals, ie every 2 to 3 hours, regardless of the sensation of need to void. Rapid contractions of the pelvic floor muscles (quick flicks) involve 2-second contractions of the pelvic floor muscles followed by sustained (endurance)

Pelvic floor muscles

A series of muscles that form a sling or hammock across the outlet of the pelvis; these muscles, together with their surrounding tissue, are responsible for keeping all of the pelvic organs (bladder, uterus, and rectum) in place and functioning correctly.

Timed or prophylactic voiding

A type of therapy that involves urinating at 2- to 3-hour intervals, no matter if there is an urge to void or not.

contractions of 5 seconds or longer with at least 10 seconds of relaxation between contractions. One should gradually increase the number of repetitions and the intensity of the contractions to a maximum of up to 60 per day, each held for 10 seconds. Performing the pelvic floor muscle contractions properly is important. Women should pull the pelvic floor up and in. Another way to help identify the pelvic floor muscles is to place a gloved finger into the vagina—the woman should feel tightening around her finger if the contraction is performed properly.

Behavioral therapy is often one of the first-line therapies used in the treatment of OAB with or without stress urinary incontinence. It may be combined with pharmacological therapy. Studies assessing the success rates of behavioral therapy and pharmacological therapy demonstrate an improved result with the combination as opposed to either therapy alone.

35. Can dietary changes affect OAB symptoms?

There are certain foods that may aggravate OAB symptoms.

- Caffeine acts as a diuretic, increasing the amount of urine that your kidneys make, which may lead to an increase in urinary frequency. Caffeine may act in certain people as a bladder irritant and thus may increase frequency and may affect urgency.
- A high intake of acidic foods may lead to a more acidic urine which may also act to irritate the bladder.
- Too much of a decreased fluid intake results in concentrated urine which may irritate the bladder.

- Artificially sweetened drinks may also have effects in some individuals on the bladder increasing urgency and frequency symptoms.

Compliance

The consistency and accuracy with which a patient follows the regimen prescribed by a physician or other healthcare professional.

36. *What is the success rate of behavioral therapy?*

Although behavioral therapy is effective, it requires motivation and **compliance**. It works only if the pelvic floor exercises are done and the dietary and lifestyle changes are adhered to. Figuring this out for yourself and altering your habits accordingly is another part of behavioral therapy. For the elderly, there is often the additional need of a dedicated caregiver to assist with therapy. The benefits of behavioral therapy are related to continuation with the therapy. Studies evaluating the durability of behavioral therapy have demonstrated initial response rates as high as 85% and 3-year response rates as high as 48%. This drop in the response rate is most likely related to a lack of continuation of the behavioral therapy regimen.

Patient satisfaction with behavioral therapy for the treatment of OAB with or without stress incontinence is high. This is reflected in the fifth National Association for Continence Survey of 130,000 members, in which 50% of patients ranked conservative therapies in general and 25% ranked pelvic floor muscle exercises specifically as "most helpful."

Some healthcare workers have reported an improvement in the frequency of incontinent episodes in as many as 80% of women with urgency and mixed incontinence treated with behavioral therapy. In one study, 96.5% of the women were happy to continue with behavioral therapy including pelvic floor muscle exercises indefinitely, and only 14% desired an alternative form of therapy. When compared to oxybutynin, behavioral therapy was associated with a greater percentage reduction in urgency incontinence episodes (84% compared to 72%). Of note, in this study, when behavioral therapy was combined with medical therapy there was an 84.5% to 88% reduction in incontinence episodes.

37. How do I tell whether I am better or not after my healthcare provider, nurse practioner, or healthcare provider's assistant placed me on a behavioral modification and medication regimen?

Your response to treatment may not be an all-or-nothing response (i.e., incontinent before starting therapy and dry once starting therapy). Typically, you will see some improvement with medical therapy within 1 to 2 weeks of starting therapy, but it may take 4 to 12 weeks to see the maximum response. Behavioral therapy also takes time. Your healthcare provider, nurse practitioner, or healthcare provider's assistant may recommend that you complete a baseline voiding diary before you start treatment and then complete a diary after a few weeks on therapy so that you can track your changes. Voiding diaries are helpful in identifying improvements in urinary frequency. Some individuals will not quantify their response but will state that they feel that they have more control. Lastly, remember that with respect to frequency of urination, it is felt that a normal number of voids is six to eight per day. Most would agree that if you see no appreciable response in 3 to 4 weeks with a particular medication, you should either increase the dose (if you are taking a two or more dose medication) or change to another agent.

38. What is a voiding diary?

A voiding diary is used to help the patient and healthcare provider understand the patient's lower urinary tract function (see Figure 9, Question 27).

Typically, the healthcare provider will ask that you complete a daily voiding diary over several days to assess your symptoms at baseline. A 3-day diary is generally considered sufficient. The diary is also helpful in the future for evaluating your response to therapy.

The voiding diary has several components. One records the volume voided and the time of each void. In addition, the number and severity of incontinence episodes and the time of such episodes are recorded. The volume of fluid and the type of fluid are also recorded. All fluid (ice cream, ices, soup, some fruits, etc.) must be included. This allows for identification of those individuals who drink excessive amounts of fluid or who have a high intake of caffeinated fluids.

Caffeine is a diuretic (stimulates the kidneys to produce increased amounts of urine) and can be a bladder irritant. Those individuals with a high fluid intake, more than 2.5 liters (2.37 quarts) per day, may benefit from decreasing their fluid intake. Similarly, highly acidic diets or overzealous intake of cranberry products, juice, or pills, may lead to an acidic urine that may irritate the bladder. Lastly, too little fluid intake causes the urine to be concentrated, and this too may irritate the bladder.

39. What is timed voiding?

Timed or prophylactic voiding is an essential component of behavioral therapy. If an individual experiences urgency every 3 hours, he/she is instructed to urinate every 2 hours to begin with. The idea is to empty the bladder before the pressure or volume is reached that would ordinarily "kick off" the urgency. With behavioral modification and (usually) medications, the intervals between voiding are gradually lengthened. For those individuals who suffer from urinary frequency they may already be voiding more frequently than this. For those individuals who suffer from urgency incontinence timed voiding will ideally also decrease the volume of urine that is lost at the time of an urgency incontinent episode. In the elderly, a caregiver may be required to prompt voiding and assist the individual with getting to and from the bathroom.

Those individuals who suffer from urgency and frequency with or without urgency incontinence are asked to try to delay voiding. With delayed voiding, the individual consciously tries to ignore or abort any sensation of bladder fullness or urgency and hold his/her urine for a progressively longer period of time to gradually increase his/her bladder capacity.

40. What are pelvic floor muscle exercises or Kegel exercises?

Developed in 1948 by Dr. Arnold Kegel, this series of exercises involve the pelvic floor muscles. Pelvic floor muscles are a group of muscles that are attached to the pelvic bone and act like a hammock to support the pelvic organs, which include the bladder, uterus, and rectum. These muscles may be weakened by childbirth, prior pelvic surgery, or obesity. **Kegel exercises** have been used in the treatment of stress urinary incontinence since the late 1940s with high cure or improvement rates up to 84% initially reported.

Kegel exercises

Exercises designed to strengthen weak pelvic floor muscles

The use of pelvic floor muscle exercises in the treatment of pure urgency incontinence and mixed urinary incontinence (urgency incontinence plus stress incontinence) is based on the observations that contraction (tightening) of the pelvic floor muscles can inhibit bladder contraction. Pelvic floor muscle exercises require a motivated, diligent, and properly instructed individual. Similar to weight lifting, strengthening of the pelvic floor muscles requires repetitive contractions of the pelvic floor muscles on a daily basis. Infrequent performance will not lead to beneficial results.

Many people find it difficult to identify the pelvic floor muscles and to contract these muscles. Typically, when an individual is asked to contract the pelvic floor muscles, the muscles of the buttocks are tightened. Actually, neither the buttock nor the thigh muscles are involved in these exercises. Placing a finger or special weight (called a vaginal cone) in the vagina (for women) or anus (for men) and contracting the muscles will produce a tightening around the finger or prevent loss of the weight if the person is in a standing position. Both are helpful strategies to identify the pelvic floor muscles. For those individuals who have a difficult time identifying the pelvic floor muscles, **biofeedback** can be used to identify them (see Question 43).

Biofeedback

Information about one or more of an individual's normally unconscious body processes is made available to the individual through a visual (see), auditory (hear), or tactile (touch) signal.

A good way to start Kegel exercises is to perform the exercises for 5 minutes twice a day. You should tighten/squeeze the pelvic floor muscles for a count of four, and then relax for a count of four, doing this repetitively for a total of 5 minutes. If you find that you cannot do this for a full 5 minutes at the start, then decrease to a tolerable time and gradually build up to 5 minutes. The exercises can be done anytime and anywhere. It is easiest to perform the exercises at the same times each day to help build a routine. Once perfected, the best results for OAB symptoms (urgency) are achieved by "quick flicks" (rapid contractions of the pelvic floor muscles) until the sensation of urgency subsides. It is best to stop all other activity and try to relax when doing these.

41. How successful are Kegel exercises?

The results of Kegel exercises will not occur immediately. Similar to weight lifting, it takes time to strengthen the pelvic floor muscles and they will only remain strong when one is regularly performing the exercises. In most women, it will take 6 to 12 weeks to notice a change in urine loss, provided that the exercises are being performed properly and regularly. Several studies have confirmed the **efficacy** of pelvic floor muscle exercises in urgency and mixed urinary incontinence. In one clinical study, the number of urgency incontinence episodes per week decreased by 80%, and the time between voiding increased from 2.13 hours to 3.44 hours with the use of pelvic floor muscle exercises.

Efficacy
Extent to which a specific intervention, procedure, regimen, or service produces a beneficial result under ideal conditions.

42. Who is a candidate for Kegel exercises?

The ideal candidate for Kegel exercises is a highly motivated individual. This person must be capable of learning the exercises and performing the exercises on his or her own. To facilitate learning, the individual must be able to understand and follow directions. In addition, he/she must realize that Kegel exercises require a commitment to long-term therapy. Kegel exercises are effective in stress, urgency, and mixed urinary incontinence, and thus in the absence of motivational and educational factors virtually everyone is a candidate for Kegel exercises.

43. What is biofeedback?

Biofeedback is a form of learning and re-education. With biofeedback, information about one or more of an individual's normally unconscious body processes is made available to the individual through a visual (see), auditory (hear), or tactile (touch) signal. Objective responses can be recorded on a tracing so the individual can review them.

When evaluating pelvic floor muscle activity, electromyography (EMG) is performed whereas a cystometrogram is used to measure and evaluate bladder muscle activity. Electromyography measures the activity of select muscles by the use of electrodes that are placed near or into the muscles. To evaluate the pelvic floor muscles, the electrodes may be placed on the skin near the anus, or special probes may be placed into the vagina, anus, or urethra. These electrodes are connected to a specialized machine that displays the activity of the muscles on a screen and records it onto a paper tracing. Relaxation of the pelvic floor muscles leads to a flat line on the tracing whereas contraction of the muscles leads to an up and down line on the tracing. The patient is then able to see when he/she is relaxing or contracting the pelvic floor muscles.

44. Who is a candidate for biofeedback?

Not all individuals will need biofeedback. Those individuals who are having trouble identifying their pelvic floor muscles or who are failing pelvic floor muscle exercises are candidates for biofeedback. As with pelvic floor muscle exercises, biofeedback requires a highly motivated individual who performs the exercises daily.

45. Is biofeedback provided in my healthcare provider's office?

In most cases biofeedback can be performed right in your healthcare provider's office. Usually a specially trained nurse, healthcare provider's assistant, or a nurse practitioner performs the biofeedback. However, in some cases the biofeedback may be performed by a physical therapist and in this situation it may be performed at a different site. Each office may use different forms of biofeedback.

46. What is the success rate of biofeedback?

The combination of behavioral therapy including Kegel exercises and biofeedback has been shown to be superior to either therapy alone. This form of therapy works better for stress urinary incontinence than urgency incontinence, however. Younger women and those without estrogen deficiency tend to do better with biofeedback than older women and women with low estrogen levels.

47. What happens if behavioral therapy and biofeedback don't work?

Often a combination of behavioral and medical (**antimuscarinics**) therapy are used as the initial treatment of OAB symptoms. Some people are started initially

Antimuscarinic

A type of medication that blocks the attachment of the neurotransmitter responsible for normal bladder contraction to the receptor on the bladder muscle cells that initiates the process of contraction when activated by the neurotransmitter acetylcholine. They also block sensory (sensation) signals from the bladder to the central nervous system.

on behavioral therapy and, if needed, biofeedback. In these individuals if the behavioral/biofeedback therapy fails then an antimuscarinic agent should be added. If one fails combination therapy, a different antimuscarinic can be tried. If two or more different antimuscarinic agents have been tried, particularly if each has been used in combination with behavioral therapy/biofeedback, then it is reasonable to consider the next step, which is typically **neuromodulation**, as it is approved by the FDA. Another alternative is the injection into the bladder muscle of botulinum toxin, which is currently an investigational therapy in the United States.

48. What medications are available to treat OAB?

There are a variety of medications that are currently approved by the Food and Drug Administration (FDA). The goal of all of these medications is the suppression of the symptoms, which will lead to less urgency, urinary frequency, and urgency incontinence episodes. Currently, antimuscarinic agents are the "gold standard" for the pharmacologic management of OAB. Historically, antimuscarinics have been demonstrated to be effective in increasing bladder capacity and inhibiting **involuntary bladder contractions/ detrusor overactivity**, however, their use has been limited due to the incidence of side effects. Since OAB is a condition that adversely affects quality of life, it is important to have a medical therapy that improves the symptoms of OAB but does not cause side effects that will have a significant negative effect on quality of life. Thus, the major emphasis on the development of new

Neuromodulation

Surgical placement of a permanent continuous nerve stimulator and its electrode wires to alter the function of the organ(s) innervated by that nerve or nerves.

Involuntary bladder contractions/ detrusor overactivity

Bladder contractions that occur during the filling/storage phase of bladder function. They may be associated with urinary frequency, urgency, and urgency incontinence.

medical therapies is on decreasing the side effect profile of the medications while maintaining efficacy. A variety of novel ways of administering drugs have been utilized to help in this endeavor. Drugs may be given in several different ways: in multiple doses per day in the traditional delivery system, the pill or capsule; in a sustained release/long-acting formulation that allows for once a day dosing; a **transdermal** (skin patch or gel) system; or as an intravesical (placed directly into the bladder) preparation.

Transdermal

Medication is delivered to the body by a skin patch or a gel.

49. How do antimuscarinics work to decrease OAB symptoms?

OAB symptoms may arise from a variety of etiologies. Historically, it was thought that antimuscarinic agents worked primarily at the level of the bladder muscle, preventing the stimulus for the bladder muscle to contract. Antimuscarinics work by blocking the attachment of the neurotransmitter, acetylcholine, that binds to the receptor in the bladder muscle cell that initiates the process of contraction (see **Figure 11**).

More recently, an additional role in the "afferent pathway" or sensory pathway (carries impulses from the bladder to the central nervous system) has been proposed. During bladder filling and stretch, nerves in the bladder lining and submucosa are stimulated and transmit messages from the bladder to the brain. Over activity in these "afferent or sensation carrying nerves," or a decrease in the ability of the brain to handle this afferent nerve activity, may lead to OAB symptoms. The antimuscarinic agents are now thought also to inhibit or dampen the sensory impulses going from the bladder to the spinal cord.

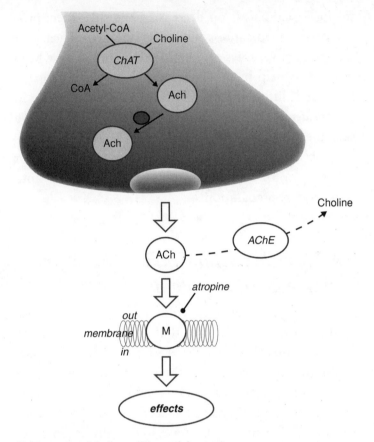

Figure 11 Acetylcholine and muscarinic receptors

There are currently five different types of muscarinic receptors.

The M3 receptors are responsible for detrusor contraction, yet they comprise only a relatively small percentage of the muscarinic receptors in the bladder (20% to 30%). When the parasympathetic nerves release acetylcholine, the chemical binds to the M3 receptor and, through a complex interaction involving calcium, the bladder muscle is stimulated to contract. M3 receptors have also been identified on the urothelium (inner lining) of the bladder and are thought to play a role in the "afferent pathway" whereby nerve impulses are transmitted from the bladder to the brain. Antimuscarinics may act to inhibit (block) both of these actions.

The M2 receptor is the most abundant receptor in the bladder (80%). Whether it has a role in normal bladder muscle activity or in certain pathologic states is a matter of debate. The actual role of the M2 receptor in human bladders is not fully understood. M2 receptors have also been identified on the urothelium (the inner lining) of the bladder and may play a role in the afferent pathway along with M3 receptors.

50. Is there anyone who should not take an antimuscarinic (anticholinergic) medication?

Antimuscarinic therapy should not be used in individuals with urinary retention, poor stomach emptying, prior allergic reaction to the medication, those with untreated narrow angle glaucoma, or anyone at risk of developing any one of these conditions. If you have glaucoma, the safest thing to do is to check with your eye healthcare provider prior to starting an antimuscarinic. Care should be taken in using antimuscarinics in individuals with liver or kidney failure. Question 55 discusses the side effects of this therapy.

51. What are the available antimuscarinics/anticholinergics?

Currently used medications in the United States for the treatment of OAB include: darifenacin (Enablex,

Novartis), fesoterodine (Toviaz, Pfizer) oxybutynin immediate release (Ditropan), oxybutynin XL (Ditropan XL), solifenacin (Vesicare, Astellas), tolterodine immediate release (Detrol IR, Pfizer), tolterodine long-acting (Detrol LA, Pfizer), transdermal oxybutynin (Oxytrol, Watson), trospium chloride (Sanctura, Indevus), and tropsium chloride extended release (Sanctura XR, Allergan). Transdermal oxybutynin (Gelnique, Watson) is the newest FDA approved antimuscarinic agent. Less commonly used medications for OAB symptoms include propantheline bromide and the **tricyclic antidepressants**. Propiverine is used in Europe but is not approved for use in the United States. All of these drugs have positive effects on the symptoms of OAB, and there is little difference between the medications in this regard. Side effect profiles may differ, common to all are dry mouth and constipation, although the tolerability varies and safety considerations do exist, which are regarded as very real by some, very hypothetical and theoretical by others.

Tricyclic antidepressants

A class of medications which may be used to treat incontinence. They lower the bladder pressure by relaxing the bladder muscle and also help further by tightening the sphincter muscle.

Oxybutynin (Ditropan IR)

Oxybutynin is one of the oldest medical therapies for OAB. Oxybutynin has been shown to act as an antimuscarinic agents with the doses used clinically to treat OAB. In the laboratory it also has direct relaxing effects on the bladder smooth muscle as a calcium antagonist and local anesthetic effects, but at drug concentrations that are far above those used clinically. Oxybutynin has more of an affinity for the M3 and M1 receptors than the M2, M4, and M5 receptors. In humans, oxybutynin has a high affinity for the salivary gland as well as the bladder muscarinic receptors which accounts for the relatively high incidence of dry mouth with immediate release oxybutynin (Ditropan).

Oxybutynin may be administered in several ways. Generic oxybutynin is often given on a three times a day basis but may be given as infrequently as once a day and as frequently as four times a day. Typically, individuals start with a 5-mg tablet on a twice a day or three times a day regimen. Generic oxybutynin has been shown to be an effective medication in the treatment of OAB. It has been shown to decrease urinary frequency, **urinary urgency**, and urgency incontinence episodes. Oxybutynin when given orally is metabolized primarily by the liver, leading to a high level of the primary metabolite, which seems responsible for most of the dry mouth reported with use.

Urinary urgency

Sudden compelling desire to urinate that often is difficult to defer.

Oxybutynin extended release (Ditropan XL)

The long-acting formulation of oxybutynin, Ditropan XL, is taken only once per day. There are several different strengths (5-mg, 10-mg, and 15-mg capsules), and it may be titrated up to 30mg per day as needed. The advantages of the once-daily dose include ease of use and a lower incidence of side effects, probably due to less liver metabolism and less active metabolite production (see Question 55). The different capsule strengths allow for flexibility and dose titration. The capsule of Ditropan XL is unique in that there is a small laser-drilled hole in the capsule. As fluid is absorbed into the capsule, the drug is pushed out of this hole in a timed fashion. The capsule itself does not break down, so don't be alarmed if you see it floating in the toilet bowl or in your colostomy bag if you have a bowel bag. This capsule should not be crushed or cut as it will no longer function as a long-acting medication. At higher doses Ditropan XL has been reported to be associated with some cognitive dysfunction in older patients.

Transdermal Oxybutynin (Oxytrol)

A newer form of delivery of oxybutynin is transdermal oxybutynin, the skin patch. The oxybutynin is contained within a thin, almost clear adhesive patch that is attached to the skin on a twice-weekly basis. The patch may be applied to the abdomen, buttock, or the hip. A new application site should be used with each new patch to avoid re-application to the same area within a 7-day period. There is no difference in the absorption of the oxybutynin when the patch is applied to different areas of the body. Each patch contains a total of 36mg of oxybutynin and releases about 4mg of oxybutynin per day through the skin. After application of the first patch, it takes 24 to 48 hours to reach the systemic level of 3mg to 4mg, and the concentration remains steady for approximately 96 hours. Thus, the patch cannot be used on an as-needed basis (called "prn"). Similar to the once-daily preparation, the patch decreases the amount of oxybutynin that is metabolized by the liver and thus decreases the amount of the active metabolite. This reduction in the amount of the active metabolite improves the tolerability by decreasing the incidence and severity of dry mouth.

Advantages of transdermal oxybutynin include its ease of use and decreased anticholinergic side effect profile compared to oxybutynin. It is reported that in 99.3% of individuals, the patch completely adheres well to the skin. In some individuals, skin irritation at the patch application site is a problem. Reports indicate that 8% develop redness at the site of patch application, and 17% develop itchiness at the site. Skin irritation may be a more significant and worrisome problem in the elderly who have thin, sensitive skin.

Transdermal Oxybutynin Gel (Gelnique)

Gelnique is the newest antimuscarinic agent and is an easy to use gel formulation of oxybutynin. It was approved by the FDA in January 2009. Individuals apply one sachet of Gelnique once daily to dry, intact skin on the abdomen, upper arms/shoulders or thighs. One should rotate the application sites. Transdermal oxybutynin gel is associated with a low incidence of side effects and a lower incidence of application site reactions than the transdermal oxybutynin patch (Oxytrol). Statistically significant improvements in overactive bladder symptoms compared to placebo have been demonstrated in the clinical trials. Because it is a topical preparation, person to person transfer-rance is possible and the application site should be covered if it will come into contact with the skin of another individual. In addition, it is recommended that one avoid bathing, swimming, showering or immersing the application site in water for one hour after application.

Tolterodine (Detrol)

Tolterodine is the first antimuscarinic medication developed solely for use in OAB. Most of the medications currently used for OAB were first developed for use for irritable bowel syndrome. Unlike oxybutynin, tolterodine is not particularly selective for a particular muscarinic receptor and, thus, it equally affects M2 and M3 receptors. Initial laboratory results suggest that it affects the bladder more than the salivary gland, and the initial publicity around the drug suggested equal efficacy to oxybutynin but fewer side effects, such as dry mouth and constipation (see Table 5). Unlike oxybutynin, the active metabolite of tolterodine shares the same properties as the parent compound. The chemical structure and molecular size of tolterodine should make it less able to penetrate the brain than oxybutynin. When brain wave function is measured by a machine known as an electroencephalograph (which produces electroencephalograms, EEGs), tolterodine is associated with fewer changes than oxybutynin. The clinical significance of these EEG changes is unknown. Tolterodine is available in two formulations, a twice-daily formulation and a once-daily formulation (Detrol LA). The usual daily dose is 2mg orally twice daily or one 4-mg Detrol LA capsule. Lower doses, 1mg orally twice daily or one 2-mg Detrol LA capsule, may be used in the elderly.

Long Acting Tolterodine (Detrol LA)

Unlike Ditropan XL, the long acting tolterodine capsule itself is not responsible for its extended release action. Rather, inside the Detrol LA capsule, there are very tiny balls (microspheres) containing the medication that provides for its continuous release throughout a 24-hour period. The advantages of the once-daily preparation include ease of use, improved compliance, and a relative stabilization of the peak (the highest amount of drug in the bloodstream) and trough (the lowest amount of drug in the bloodstream prior to taking the next dose) levels of the drug in the patient's bloodstream. The decrease in the peak level may account for its better side effect profile when compared to the twice-daily formulation. The increase in the trough may account for a slightly better result (efficacy) for the extended release preparation. Detrol LA has been shown to improve urgency incontinence and urgency, allowing an increasing number of individuals to finish tasks before going to the bathroom when the symptom of urgency does occur.

Trospium Chloride

Trospium chloride (Sanctura) is an antimuscarinic that has been used in Europe for the management of OAB symptoms for over 30 years. Trospium chloride's chemical structure is such that it is unlikely to penetrate the brain and thus does not appear to affect cognitive function. Trospium chloride is usually administered orally twice a day in 20mg. Trospium chloride should be taken 1 hour before meals or on an empty stomach. It is not well absorbed if taken with food. An advantage of this medication is that it has little potential interaction with other medications.

Trospium Chloride Extended Release (Sanctura XR)

A long acting form of Trospium chloride (Sanctura XR) is also available for the treatment of OAB. The recommended dose is 60mg once per day and, as with trospium chloride, it should be taken 1 hour prior to a meal or on an empty stomach. Trospium chloride extended release is excreted intact by the kidneys with essentially none of the drug metabolized by the liver. Drug-drug interactions are therefore not anticipated with this medication. The effect of trospium chloride extended release on other drugs excreted by the kidneys is not well known. Studies looking at the effect of co-administration with digoxin (a heart medication that is secreted by the kidneys) did not show an effect on the metabolism of either drug. Trospium chloride extended release has a lower incidence of side effects compared to the immediate release formulation.

Solifenacin (Vesicare)

Solifenacin (Vesicare) is another antimuscarinic, approved by the FDA for use in OAB. It appears to have a tissue preference for the bladder over the salivary gland. It is a once-daily oral medication and is available in two doses, 5mg and 10mg. Unlike many of the other anticholinergics, solifenacin has a long half-life which may cause it to take a little longer to show a positive effect than the other drugs but only by a couple of days. Solifenacin shows a similar efficacy to oxybutynin and tolterodine. The company was the first to emphasize the importance of reduction of urgency and "dry days," reporting the percent of patients with urgency incontinence who remained dry for 3 consecutive days. Whether solifenacin is able to penetrate the brain is unknown at present. Reports of cognitive dysfunction are few. The tablet cannot be crushed or cut.

Darifenacin (Enablex)

Darifenacin (Enablex) is an antimuscarinic agent that is relatively selective for the M3 receptor. This muscarinic receptor is the receptor primarily responsible for normal bladder contractility. Darifenacin is available in two, once-daily doses, 7.5mg and 15mg, which will allow for dose titration and dose flexibility. Several cognitive function studies have been performed with darifenacin and none have shown an effect on cognitive function including memory. In one animal model, darifenacin was shown to have more affinity for the bladder than the salivary gland. Its relative M3 receptor selectivity prevents it from having an effect on the heart rate, and it does not affect electrical conduction within the heart. The efficacy of darifenacin is similar to that of the other approved antimuscarinics. The tablet cannot be crushed or cut.

Propiverine

Propiverine is an orally administered agent which, like oxybutynin, has a number of reported actions but which probably functions as an antimuscarinic when used in the commonly prescribed doses. It is typically given as a 15mg-tablet twice a day. Studies comparing propiverine 15mg-po BID to tolterodine 2mg-po BID demonstrated a similar efficacy between the two drugs. The side effects of propiverine are similar to the other antimuscarinics. Propiverine is not available for use in the United States.

Fesoterodine (Toviaz)

Fesoterodine is an antimuscarinic agent that was approved for use in the United States in November 2008. It was approved for use in Europe in 2008. It is very similar in chemical structure to tolterodine. Fesoterodine is rapidly broken down to essentially the same active metabolite as that of tolterodine. The rapid and complete initial metabolism is said to provide for a more consistent level of active metabolite in all individuals. It is available in two doses, 4mg and 8mg, to be taken once a day.

Propantheline Bromide

Propantheline bromide is a nonselective antimuscarinic that is usually given orally four times a day in doses of 15mg to 30mg. Each individual may require a different dose, so it is recommended that you titrate to the dose that produces the desired results with tolerable side effects. Some individuals will require even higher doses to achieve an acceptable response. Individual responses vary, and a review of five randomized controlled studies demonstrated that the use of propantheline bromide decreased urgency by 0% to 53%. Propantheline bromide is rarely obtainable in the United States.

Antidepressants

Some antidepressants have been utilized in the treatment of OAB. Imipramine (Tofranil) is the antidepressant whose use is most commonly reported. The data is sketchy and it is not entirely clear how imipramine actually would affect OAB symptoms. It does possess antimuscarinic properties outside of the bladder, and it prevents the reuptake of two neurotransmitters in the brain and spinal cord: serotonin and noradrenaline. Both serotonin and noradrenaline are involved in the complex interactions related to normal bladder filling and emptying. Dosing of imipramine varies. *Imipramine can have significant toxic effects on the cardiovascular system,* including abnormal heart rhythms and lowering of the blood pressure, when going from a sitting to a standing position (called **orthostatic hypotension**), and abnormal heart rhythms. Thus, it should be kept in a location that is not accessible to younger children. If the patient wishes to discontinue imipramine after a prolonged period of use, it is important to wean off the medication under a healthcare provider's supervision as opposed to stopping it suddenly.

Orthostatic hypotension

Lowering of blood pressure while moving from a sitting or supine position to a standing position; potential for dizziness and collapsing.

52. How do these medications compare with respect to efficacy?

All of the currently approved antimuscarinic agents have been demonstrated to be effective in reducing the symptoms of OAB. Overall, the medications have a similar efficacy. There is a lack of well-designed comparative studies which would enable us to determine if one medication is significantly superior to another with respect to efficacy. Some of the medications are available in more than one dose, which allows increasing the dose in individuals who do not achieve adequate efficacy but have minimal side effects.

53. If one medication does not work, does that mean that all of them are going to fail?

If one medication does not prove to be effective enough, that does not mean that all of the other available antimuscarinic agents are going to fail. If you tried one that is available only in a single dose (Oxytrol, Sanctura, Sanctura XR, and Detrol LA 4mg) then it may make sense to try a different one that has more

Treatment of Overactive Bladder

than one dose available. If the medication is working adequately but the side effects are bothersome, then it would be best to choose another drug to see if fewer side effects are experienced. If you have failed to respond to several of the antimuscarinics at a high dose and you have altered your lifestyle somewhat then it is probably best to look at alternative forms of therapy as opposed to trying every one of the antimuscarinics available. If you do not respond adequately to one medication, this does not mean that the other medications won't work for you. It is not unreasonable to try an alternative antimuscarinic agent prior to proceeding to other forms of treatment.

54. How do these medications compare with respect to doses available, the half life (the time it takes for half of the drug to clear from your system), and how they are broken down?

Table 4   Dosing, half-life and metabolism rate of OAB medications

Medication	Dose	Half-life, hrs	Metabolism
DARIFENACIN			
Darifenacin (Enablex)	7.5-15mg Once daily	7.4-19.95 hrs	Liver
FESOTERODINE			
Fesoterodine	4mg 8mg Once daily	7.3 hrs 8.59 hrs	Liver
OXYBUTYNIN			
Oxybutynin IR (Ditropan)	5mg Three times a day	4 hrs	Liver

Table 4   Continued

Medication	Dose	Half-life, hrs	Metabolism
Oxybutynin ER (Ditropan XL)	5-30mg Once daily	12 hrs	Liver
Suspension	5mg Three times a day	4 hrs	Liver
Transdermal patch (Oxytrol)	3.9mg/day Apply twice a week	NA	Liver
Transdermal oxybutynin gel (Gelnique)	1g 100mg/g/day (1.14 mL)	64 hrs at a steady state. Steady state concentration is reached within 7 days of continuous doing.	Liver

SOLIFENACIN

Solifenacin (Vesicare)	5-10mg Once daily	45-68 hrs	Liver

TOLTERODINE

Tolterodine IR (Detrol)	1-2mg Twice a day	2.2-9.6 hrs	Liver
Tolterodine ER (Detrol LA)	2-4mg Once daily	8 hrs	Liver

TROSPIUM CHLORIDE

Trospium Chloride IR (Sanctura)	20mg Twice a day	20 hrs	No liver metabolism Ester hydrolysis Renal excretion
Trospium Chloride ER (Sanctura XR)	60mg Once daily	35 hrs	No liver metabolism Ester hydrolysis Renal excretion

55. What are the side effects of antimuscarinics?

Muscarinic receptors are located throughout the body including the salivary gland, the bowel, the heart, and the brain (see **Figure 12**).

Thus, an antimuscarinic agent used for the treatment of OAB has the potential of affecting other areas throughout the body. The more common side effects related to antimuscarinic agents include dry mouth and constipation. Less common side effects include blurred vision, facial flushing, problems with **cognition** (memory, learning, and thinking), and, rarely, urinary retention (the inability to urinate).

Cognition

General term encompassing thinking, learning, and memory.

- Dry mouth: The salivary glands contain M1 and M3 receptors, so antimuscarinic agents affect salivary production. Baseline salivary production, that is, the production of saliva at times during the day when

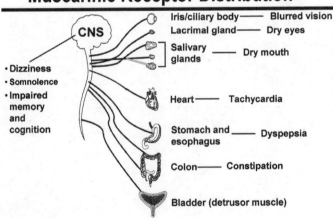

Figure 12   Muscarinic receptor locations throughout the body

From Abrams P, Wein AJ: The Overactive Bladder: A Widespread and Treatable Condition. Reprinted with permission from Eric Sparre Medical AB.

one is not eating, is affected by antimuscarinics. It is this constant salivary production that coats our teeth and gums and maintains our dental health. Saliva is also produced when one eats or drinks something. This eating-induced salivary production is not disturbed by antimuscarinics. Dry mouth makes it more difficult to chew and swallow food, makes the oral tissues (gums and tongue) more prone to infection, increases the risk of tooth decay, and makes it more difficult to taste salty, bitter, sweet, and sour flavors. There are a variety of treatments available for dry mouth (see Question 60).

- Constipation: There are muscarinic receptors in the colon (M3) that govern its ability to contract and propel stool through it. Methods to improve bowel function while on an antimuscarinic include adequate fluid intake, increased fiber intake, and the use of stool softeners and stimulants/laxatives as needed. For those individuals prone to constipation, it is very helpful to get your bowels regular before starting the antimuscarinic therapy (see Questions 58 and 59).

- Central nervous system: The brain contains muscarinic receptors, but unlike many areas of the body, the brain has a protective barrier called the **blood brain barrier (BBB)**. This semipermeable barrier prevents a variety of substances, including many medications, from entering the brain. Thus, the ability of an antimuscarinic to cause central nervous system side effects is governed by its ability to cross this blood brain barrier and to affect particular receptors. Antimuscarinics that are able to cross the blood brain barrier and affect M1 receptors in the brain may affect one's cognition (thinking, learning, and memory).

Blood brain barrier (BBB)

Semipermeable network of the tiniest blood vessels called capillaries with special endothelial cells surrounding the brain; the barrier prevents a variety of agents such as medications from passing through and entering the brain. Its function is to protect the brain from potentially harmful substances (like certain medications), other neurotransmitters, and hormones in the body, and to maintain the brain in a constant environment.

- Urinary retention: Although the antimuscarinics have been shown to decrease involuntary contractions and increase bladder capacity, they rarely cause urinary retention. In the absence of significant obstruction to the outflow of urine, it does not appear that in general antimuscarinic medications used only in the recommended dosages cause or worsen voiding difficulties. Studies of women on antimuscarinics have demonstrated no increase in the number of urinary tract infections, no slow stream, and no increase in the amount of urine left in the bladder after voiding (post-void residual) or changes in the force of urination. In men, an antimuscarinic (tolterodine) given for 1 month to individuals with bladder outlet obstruction did not make their voiding worse. In men with OAB and no signs or symptoms to suggest obstruction (generally younger men), antimuscarinics are often used alone. In men with, or suspected of having, bladder outlet obstruction, secondary to prostatic enlargement, the prostatic component is generally treated first. If the OAB symptoms persist and are bothersome, an antimuscarinic agent is added.

Side effects of these drugs are due to their effects on areas in the body other than the bladder.

The use of a dosing regimen several times a day is often associated with high (peak) and low (trough) levels of drug throughout the dosing period. The high levels of drug may be associated with more side effects, whereas the low levels may affect the efficacy of the drug. Thus, the use of a once-daily preparation, through a sustained release delivery system, allows for a steady amount of drug in the bloodstream throughout the day. This avoidance of peak and trough drug levels helps to decrease the side effects and maximize the benefits of the medication.

Drugs are broken down (metabolized) via different organs in the body. The most common organ involved in drug metabolism is the liver. For a variety of drugs, including many of the drugs used for OAB, the metabolism of the drug by the liver results in a chemical (metabolite) that can also work on the condition, but it can cause side effects that may be similar, worse, or less than the original medication. For those drugs where the metabolite is associated with worse side effects, it is important to develop a way to give the medication to minimize its metabolism by the liver. In doing so, there will be less of the metabolite and more of the original drug around, and thus fewer side effects. There are three ways to accomplish this task. One is to use a slow release capsule that allows for much of the drug to bypass the liver because it is absorbed lower down in the bowel, in an area where the circulation does not directly pass to the liver. The second is to use a skin patch which allows the drug to go directly into the circulation, and the third is to place the drug directly into the bladder. All of these ways of administering the drug help to decrease any metabolism by the liver. Finally, since many organ systems throughout the body have muscarinic receptors, it would be advantageous to have a drug that is more selective for the particular organ that is being treated, ie the bladder in the case of OAB. A bladder-selective drug would have a greater effect on the bladder than other organ systems.

56. How common are the side effects with each of these medications?

The reported side effects for each of these medications are based on placebo controlled studies and thus cannot be used for direct comparison. In addition, during the various clinical trials the incidence of side effects in individuals taking a placebo varied significantly thus making it even more difficult to directly compare the different results. **Table 5** lists the reported incidence of side effects for each of the agents as well as the placebo in the large studies performed to gain FDA approval. Drug to placebo ratios are also listed. For information on drug to placebo ratios see Question 57.

57. I hear my healthcare providers talking about placebos. What is a placebo and what is a placebo response?

A placebo is a tablet, liquid, or other form of medication, that actually contains no active ingredients. It is often referred to as a "sugar pill." Placebos are used in clinical studies evaluating new medications to determine whether the new medication is effective. In these studies, patients are randomized (like the flip of a coin) into two groups, one that receives a placebo and the other that receives the new medication that is being evaluated. The medication and the placebo are disguised so that they look alike and neither the patient nor the healthcare provider is aware of which one of the two the patient is receiving. This is called a double-blind study. It is expected that if the drug is effective, patients randomized to the new medication will have a better response than those randomized to the placebo.

Table 5   Side effects of drugs used to treat OAB

Drug	Adverse Reaction	Drug AE%	Placebo AE%	Drug to Placebo ratio
Darifenacin (Enablex) 7.5 mg	Dry mouth	20.2%	8.2%	2.5
	Constipation	14.8%	6.2%	2.4
	Dizziness	0.9%	1.3%	0.7
15mg	Dry mouth	35.3%	8.2%	4.3
	Constipation	21.3%	6.2%	3.4
	Dizziness	2.1%	1.3%	1.6
Fesoterodine (Toviaz) 4mg	Dry mouth	18.8%	7.0%	2.7
	Constipation	4.2%	2.0%	2.1
	Insomnia	1.3%	0.5%	2.6
8mg	Dry mouth	34.6%	7.0%	4.9
	Constipation	6.0%	2.0%	3.0
	Insomnia	0.4%	0.5%	0.8
Solifenacin (Vesicare) 5mg	Dry mouth	10.9%	4.2%	2.6
	Constipation	5.4%	2.9%	1.9
	Dizziness	1.9%	1.8%	1.1
	Blurred vision	3.8%	1.8%	2.1
10mg	Dry mouth	27.6%	4.2%	6.6
	Constipation	13.4%	2.9%	4.6
	Dizziness	1.8%	1.8%	1.0
	Blurred vision	4.8%	1.8%	2.7
Tolterodine LA 4mg (Detrol LA 4mg)	Dry mouth	23 %	8 %	2.9
	Constipation	6 %	4 %	1.5
	Headache	6 %	4 %	1.5
	Dizziness	2 %	1 %	2.0
	Abnormal vision	1 %	0 %	
Transdermal oxybutynin gel (Gelnique)	Dry mouth	7.5%	2.8%	2.7
	Constipation	1.3%	0	
	Dizziness	2.8%	1.0%	2.8
Transdermal oxybutynin (Oxytrol)	Dry mouth	9.6%	8.3%	1.2
	Constipation	3.3%	0	
	Application site Pruritis	16.8%	6.1%	2.8
	Application site erythema	5.6%	2.3%	2.4
Trospium chloride IR (Sanctura)	Dry mouth	20.1%	5.8%	3.5
	Constipation	9.6%	4.6%	2.1
	Headache	4.2%	2.0%	2.1
Trospium chloride XR (Santura XR)	Dry mouth	10.7%	3.7%	2.9
	Constipation	8.5%	1.5%	5.7
	Dry eyes	1.6%	0.2%	8.0

Treatment of Overactive Bladder

87

Placebo effect occurs when a significant number of patients receiving the placebo have a change in their condition, despite not getting any actual medication. Placebo effects are usually positive, maybe surprisingly so, but rarely can be negative.

In studies evaluating OAB medications there tends to be a high placebo effect for the efficacy parameters. Part of this is attributed to the fact that patients are made more aware of their bladder condition by participation in the study. These studies usually require patients to keep bladder diaries which are a form of behavioral therapy and education.

In an effort to compare the efficacy results and side effects of drugs that have not been compared directly in studies, some healthcare providers have argued that looking at the drug to placebo response for some parameters (drug response divided by placebo response) is the best way to compare data from different studies. (Table 5) The best way to gain comparative data, however, would be through head to head studies, which are clinical studies designed to compare two or more drugs in the same study.

58. My healthcare provider asked me if I am constipated. What is the definition of constipation?

The term constipation often refers to different symptoms for different individuals and means different things to different people. Constipation is common in older adults. The estimated prevalence ranges from 2% to 28% and increases with age. Women more commonly experience constipation than men. Classification systems have been developed to define constipation. One such system is the Rome II. According to this system, chronic constipation in adults is defined as having two or more of the following for at least 12 weeks in the preceding 12 months:

- Straining with greater than 25% of bowel movements
- Lumpy or hard stools in more than 25% of bowel movements
- Sensation of incomplete bowel emptying in more than 25% of bowel movements
- Sensation of anorectal obstruction or blockage in 25% of bowel movements
- Manual maneuvers (digital evacuation, pressure on one's perineum) to facilitate passage of stools in more than 25% of bowel movements
- Less than three bowel movements per week

59. If I am prone to constipation, will these medications make it worse?

It is possible that use of an antimuscarinic agent may make your constipation worse. Blocking muscarinic receptors in the intestine, particularly the M3 receptor, can slow down the motility of the colon leading to a change in your bowel habits or constipation. All of the medications used to treat OAB have this risk, but some more so than others, and you should mention this to your healthcare provider so that the most tolerable medication may be selected.

If you are prone to constipation, it is helpful to start a bowel regimen before or at the time you start antimuscarinic therapy for your OAB symptoms. This decreases the likelihood of experiencing troubles with constipation. A bowel regimen consists of one or more of the following:

- Ensure adequate fluid intake.
- Increase fiber intake. The recommended fiber intake is 20 to 35 grams of fiber per day. Foods that are high in fiber include: fruits, vegetables, nuts, and bran. A variety of cereals are high in fiber and there are also a variety of supplement bars that are high in fiber. It is recommended that one should increase fiber by 5 grams a day each week until one reaches the recommended daily amount. If fiber is increased too quickly it may cause excessive gas and bloating.
- Take the time to have a bowel movement. There is a normal reflex, the gastrocolic reflex, that occurs when you eat a meal. When food enters the stomach, the stomach sends nerve impulses to the colon stimulating it to contract and evacuate stool. Thus, the best time to try to move your bowels is about 30 minutes after a meal. The bowels are more active in the morning, thus the best time to try to move your bowels is in the morning after breakfast. Increasing physical activity helps promote regular bowel function.
- Laxatives. There are a variety of laxatives available that work in different ways. Some work to increase stool mass and soften the stool such as psyllium (Metamucil), methylcellulose (Citrucel), and polycarbonil (Fibercon). Stimulant laxatives such as senna and bisacodyl act to increase intestinal motility and the secretion of water into the bowel. Emollient laxatives/stool softeners (docusate, Colace) allow water to enter the bowel more easily. These tend to not be as effective in patients with chronic constipation as the bulk laxatives. Lastly, osmotic laxatives,

magnesium hydroxide (milk of magnesia, MOM), oral magnesium citrate, sodium biphosphate (Phospha-Soda), sorbitol, lactulose, and polyethylene glycol cause secretion of water into the intestine. Enemas are useful if significant constipation is present but are not ideal as maintenance treatment.

60. What can I do to treat dry mouth?

The technical term for dry mouth is xerostomia and it is most often associated with decreased production of saliva by the salivary glands. Xerostomia affects more than 10% of individuals in the United States and about 25% of individuals are 65 years of age and older. There are three major salivary glands: the parotid gland, the submandibular gland, and the sublingual gland. In addition to these three there are hundreds of minor salivary glands that contribute to salivary production. The salivary glands contain M1 and M3 receptors, so antimuscarinic agents can affect salivary production. Baseline salivary production, that is, the production of saliva at times during the day when one is not eating, is affected by antimuscarinics. It is this constant salivary production that coats our teeth and gums and maintains our dental health. Saliva is also produced when one eats or drinks something. This eating-induced salivary production is not disturbed by antimuscarinics. Dry mouth makes it more difficult to chew and swallow food, makes the oral tissues (gums and tongue) more prone to infection, increases the risk of tooth decay, and makes it more difficult to taste salty, bitter, sweet, and sour flavors.

The most common causes of xerostomia are systemic medical diseases and side effects of medical treatments. A variety of major drug classes are associated with dry mouth including: antianxiety medications, antimuscarinic agents, antidepressants, antidiarrheals, antihypertensives, antihistamines, diuretics, sedatives, decongestants, bronchodilators, and anti-Parkinson's drugs as well as other medications.

Treatments for dry mouth include: frequent sips of water, drinking milk, use of olive oil to moisten your mouth, sugar-free gum and other sugar-free candies, avoiding drinks with caffeine or alcohol, avoiding smoking, and the use of a humidifier at night. Artificial saliva may be helpful as well as lubricating and hydrating creams and ointments. There are a variety of oral rinses, gels, lozenges, sprays, and mouthwashes developed to help treat dry mouth. Antiseptics may be helpful in keeping the mouth clean and in decreasing the number of bacteria that cause tooth decay and gum disease. Glycerin and lemon mouthwash can be used to try to stimulate saliva production, but these should be used sparingly as too frequent use can cause tooth decay and gum disease. Use of high concentration fluoride toothpastes may also be helpful in preventing tooth decay.

If you are experiencing bothersome dry mouth with a particular antimuscarinic let your healthcare provider know. The risk of developing dry mouth varies between the different antimuscarinics and in different individuals. Your healthcare provider may prescribe an alternative anticholinergic with a lower incidence of dry mouth.

61. Do I have to worry about interactions between an antimuscarinic medication and other medications that I am taking, so-called drug-drug interactions?

Many people with OAB symptoms have other medical problems and are on multiple medications. In general, antimuscarinic agents are safe when combined with other medications, however, there is the potential for drug-drug interactions with some of the antimuscarinic agents.

Additive Effects

Side effects of anticholinergic agents taken for OAB symptoms can be increased when taken with other medications that have similar side effects. An example would be taking an antimuscarinic agent along with a tricyclic antidepressant such as imipramine (Tofranil) or an antihistamine such as diphenhydramine (Benadryl). Particularly worrisome is the potential for increased cognitive effects, especially in the older patient, whose metabolism may be slower.

Metabolism-related Side Effects

Many drugs are metabolized by the liver, by a set of enzymes called the cytochrome P450 systems. Drugs may be metabolized by the liver to both active products or inactive products. Drugs may affect metabolism of other drugs in a variety of ways. A drug (for example, drug A) may act as an "inhibitor" when it competes with another drug (for example, drug B) for a particular enzyme, thus affecting the optimal level of metabolism of drug B, which may affect the individual's response to drug B. Such "inhibitor" drugs are classified into strong, moderate, and weak depending on how significantly they compete with other drugs for the particular enzyme. Drugs may also act as "inducers" of liver enzymes. An inducer stimulates production of the enzyme which increases the rate of metabolism of other drugs metabolized by the enzyme. By increasing the rate of metabolism of other drugs, the efficacy of the drug may be negatively affected due to its rapid breakdown. Lastly, some people genetically have poorer functioning enzymes, "poor metabolizers," and these individuals tend to have higher levels of drug in their blood stream for those drugs that are metabolized by the poorly functioning enzymes.

All currently used antimuscarinic drugs for OAB, with the exception of trospium chloride, are primarily metabolized in the liver, some preparations more so than others. Trospium chloride is primarily excreted by the kidneys into the urine.

Dosing recommendations exist for many of the OAB medications when used in conjunction with other medications that are strong inhibitors of the cytochrome P450 system.

1. The dose of darifenacin (Enablex, Novartis) should not exceed 7.5mg when individuals are taking strong inhibitors such as ketoconazole, itraconazole, ritonavir, nefinavir, clarithryomycin, and nefazadone. In patients with liver impairment the dose of Enablex should not exceed 7.5mg in patients with moderate liver impairment, and it is not recommended for use in patients with severe hepatic

impairment. Caution should be taken when darifenacin is used concomitantly with medications that are predominantly metabolized by the CYP2D6 system and which have a narrow therapeutic window, such as flecainide, thioridazine, and tricyclic antidepressants.

2. The dose of fesoterodine (Toviaz, Pfizer) should not be increased above 4mg in patients with severe renal impairment or in patients taking ketoconazole or other medications that inhibit the metabolism of fesoterodine such as clarithromycin and itraconazole. Fesoterodine is contraindicated in patients with severe liver impairment. It is contraindicated in patients with moderate to severe liver or renal impairment who are taking concomitant potent CYP3A4 inhibitors such as ketoconazole.

3. Only 5mg of solifenacin (Vesicare, Astellas) should be used in individuals on ketoconazole or other strong inhibitors as noted above. In patients with liver impairment one should not exceed 5mg, and it is not recommended for use in patients with severe hepatic impairment.

4. With tolterodine (Detrol LA, Pfizer) the dose should be decreased to 2mg once a day in individuals with significantly decreased liver function as well as in patients with significantly decreased renal function. In patients receiving ketoconazole or other potent CYP3A4 inhibitors such as certain antifungals (itraconazole, miconazole), macrolide antibiotics (erythromycin, clarithromycin), or cyclosporine or vinblastine the recommended dose of Detrol LA is 2mg per day.

5. There are no dose adjustments needed when taking trospium chloride (Sanctura, Sanctura XR, Allergan) because it is not metabolized significantly by the

liver. Theoretically, there could be interactions with other medications excreted by the kidneys, but none have been identified to date. Caution is advised regarding the use of Sanctura XR in patients with moderate to severe hepatic impairment.

6. No specific drug-drug interactions have been performed with transdermal oxybutynin gel (Gelnique, Watson). There is no experience with renal or hepatic impairment.

62. Are there other medications under investigation for use in treating OAB symptoms?

There are a variety of medications that are currently in various stages of investigation.

1. YM 178 (Astellas) is a beta-3 adrenergic receptor agonist (activates beta-3 receptors). Beta-3 receptors are found in the bladder muscle and are thought to be important in bladder relaxation. It is currently in phase II clinical trials. Other beta-3 agonists being studied include KUC-7483 (Boehringer Ingelheim) which is in phase I trials and MN-246 (Medici-Nova) also in phase I trials.

2. Neurokinin (NK)-1 receptor antagonists (blockers)-NK1 receptors are located in the spinal cord and in the nerves that control the bladder. These nerves are involved in the impulse that initiates the bladder contraction in OAB. Three are currently being evaluated: Casopitant (GSK), SSR 240600 (Sanofi-Aventis), and TA-5538 (Tanabe) in phase II trials.

For a drug to be approved by the FDA it must be studied in various rigorous clinical trials.

Phase I

This is first phase of testing in humans. These studies are designed to evaluate safety, tolerability, and pharmacodynamics (what effects a variety of given doses of drug cause) of the drug. These studies include dose-ranging so that the appropriate dose can be identified.

Phase II

These studies are performed in a larger number of patients to see how well the drug works and whether it has any tolerability or safety issues.

Phase III

These studies are randomized controlled (drug matched against placebo or another drug) multicenter (done at not one but a number of sites throughout the country or world) trials involving a large number of patients and are aimed at being the definitive assessment of whether the drug effect is greater than placebo and how effective the drug is compared to the current "gold standard" treatment.

Phase IV

These are post-marketing studies which occur after the drug is FDA-approved and being used by patients.

63. What are capsaicin and resiniferatoxin (RTX)?

Capsaicin and resiniferatoxin are agents that are used to desensitize the bladder to certain stimuli. Neither is FDA approved for treatment of OAB. Both are

Capsaicin
The active ingredient found in chili peppers; may be instilled into the bladder to decrease bladder activity.

instilled into the bladder as a liquid. They both cause an initial stimulation and inflammation, capsaicin much more so than resiniferatoxin.

Capsaicin is the active ingredient found in chili peppers. Resiniferatoxin is a chemical derived from a cactus-like plant, Euphorbia resinifera. Resiniferatoxin is roughly 100 times more potent than capsaicin but initially less irritating to the bladder. How "hot" are these chemicals? The spice industry uses a scale, called the Scoville scale, to compare pepper strengths in heat units. Bell peppers are barely a 1 on the Scoville scale, whereas pure capsaicin has a score of 16 million and resiniferatoxin a score of 16 billion Scoville heat units. Thus, both capsaicin and resiniferatoxin are very hot.

64. How do capsaicin and resiniferatoxin work?

Inside the bladder there are two types of nerves that travel from the bladder to the central nervous system. These nerves are responsible for transmitting signals of bladder fullness and/or discomfort from the bladder to the brain. One type of nerve, the small A delta fiber, transmits signals regarding bladder fullness, and nerves called C fibers detect noxious signals and initiate painful sensations. C fibers are typically excited when there is an irritation and/or infection of the bladder. When stimulated, these C fibers can facilitate or cause voiding.

When placed into the bladder, both capsaicin and resiniferatoxin cause an intense initial stimulation of the C fibers. This intense stimulation causes the nerves to run out of neurotransmitters, so they cannot transmit messages to the brain and spinal cord that would cause the sensation of urgency and bladder to contract. Because there is no permanent damage to the nerves, the therapy is reversible, but, if used as treatment, needs to be repeated periodically. However, it does take the nerves a fair amount of time to build up a new supply of neurotransmitters.

When placed into the bladder of an awake individual with normal sensation, capsaicin causes significant discomfort. In fact, it is far too uncomfortable to do this procedure without the use of either a general or spinal anesthesia. Resiniferatoxin, although it is more potent than capsaicin, does not require anesthesia because there is no intense pain when it is placed into the bladder.

65. How effective are capsaicin and resiniferatoxin? How are they administered and how long will the response last?

In a review of several studies using capsaicin to treat OAB from a variety of causes, it appeared that capsaicin was effective in decreasing bladder over activity. Studies showed that it was more effective in individuals with OAB from a neurogenic cause, such as that related to a spinal cord injury or multiple sclerosis, etc. It is less effective in individuals with OAB due to a non-neurologic cause, that is, those with hypersensitive bladders and individuals with pelvic pain. Some clinical studies with resiniferatoxin suggest that it produces clinical improvement in individuals with OAB of both neurologic and non-neurologic causes. There is still disagreement, however, as to the clinical efficacy of resiniferatoxin.

Most of the studies using resiniferatoxin have been short-term studies. Unlike capsaicin, there did not appear to be a transient worsening of the patient's symptoms after resiniferatoxin instillation. With resiniferatoxin, the results were often noted as soon as one day after the treatment, and in those who responded the response lasted for at least 3 months, the longest time that was evaluated.

Neither capsaicin nor resiniferatoxin are currently approved for routine clinical intravesical use. Capsaicin is rarely used. These medications should be administered by a healthcare provider who is familiar with their use and who has achieved the approval of the local institutional review board and regulatory authorities.

Resiniferatoxin does not cause the bladder pain that capsaicin does and, thus, it can be administered in the clinic. Since resiniferatoxin is much more potent than capsaicin, a lower dose can be used. The recommended concentration of resiniferatoxin is not yet clearly defined. Studies have used concentrations that have ranged from 1 nM (nanomole) to 10 μM (micromole). Resiniferatoxin is usually dissolved in 10% ethanol and is placed into the bladder in a similar volume and duration as capsaicin.

66. What are the side effects of capsaicin and resiniferatoxin?

Temporary worsening of urinary symptoms can occur for a few weeks after capsaicin use. Symptoms may include suprapubic (above the pubic bone) and perineal (relating to the perineum) pain, burning sensation, urinary frequency, urinary incontinence, and hematuria (presence of red blood cells in the urine). Urinary tract infections may occur as a result of catheterization with either capsaicin or resiniferatoxin use. If the capsaicin or resiniferatoxin leaks onto the skin, it may cause local skin irritation.

In those individuals with a spinal cord injury and a condition called autonomic dysreflexia, there is a risk of causing **hypertension**. These individuals should have the procedure performed under anesthesia with continuous blood pressure monitoring. These individuals should be monitored closely and have a Foley **catheter** for several days after the procedure.

67. What is botulinum toxin?

Botulinum neurotoxin is one of the most poisonous biological chemicals known. It is a chemical that is produced by the bacterium Clostridium botulinum. Very small amounts of systemic botulinum toxin can lead to paralysis. This may result from clostridial infection of the intestines, a wound, or eating food that is contaminated by Clostridium botulinum. The Clostridium botulinum bacteria produce a variety of types of botulinum toxin. The toxin that has been used most commonly in medicine is the botulinum toxin type A. All of the different types of botulinum toxin, when injected into a muscle, produce a weakening and lack of activity of the affected muscles. Botulinum toxin injection is more commonly used for cosmetic purposes (ie direct injection to remove forehead wrinkles).

Hypertension

Transitory or sustained elevated arterial blood pressure. Untreated, it can cause cardiovascular damage.

Catheter

A tube usually made of latex or silicone especially designed to be passed through the urethra into the bladder to drain the bladder.

Botulinum neurotoxin

One of the most poisonous biologic chemicals known; produced by the bacterium Clostridium botulinum; very small amounts can lead to paralysis.

68. How does botulinum toxin work in OAB?

Botulinum has been shown to prevent the release of the neurotransmitter, acetylcholine, and probably other neurotransmitters, from nerves (see **Figure 13**).

In the case of OAB, it is the release of acetylcholine from the parasympathetic neuron that results in the stimulus for the bladder muscle to contract. When the release of acetylcholine is prevented, there is no stimulus for bladder muscle contraction. It is also thought to interfere with the generation and transmission of sensory stimuli from the bladder to the central nervous system. For the toxin to be effective it must be injected directly into the bladder muscle. The bladder is readily accessible through the **cystoscope**. The cystoscope, a long telescope-like instrument, is passed through the urethra into the bladder. After inspection of the bladder, the bladder muscle is injected with the botulinum toxin through a slender hollow needle that is passed through the cystoscope into the wall of the bladder. Because the toxin only works locally and does not diffuse through the muscle of the bladder, multiple injections, typically in the range of 30 to 40, using very small amounts of the toxin, are performed during the procedure.

The botulinum toxin does not produce a permanent change in the bladder muscle, and typically its effects will last for around 3 to 9 months. Therefore, patients will generally need repeat injections over the course of time.

Cystoscope

A long telescope-like instrument that is passed through the urethra into the bladder for diagnostic and therapeutic purposes. It allows one to visualize inside the bladder and urethra.

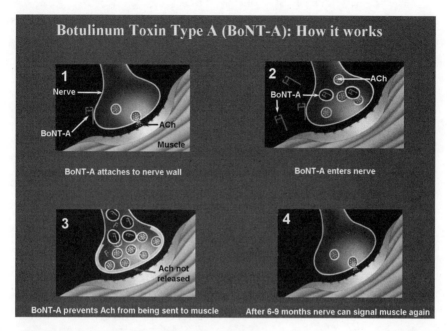

Figure 13   Botulinum toxin Type A (BoNT-A): How It Works

Courtesy of Allergan Inc., Irvine, California.

69. How effective is botulinum toxin in OAB?

Botulinum toxin bladder injection has been safely used in clinical trials in individuals with OAB as a result of spinal cord injury who have failed maximal medical therapy. In such individuals, an improvement in the number of incontinence episodes and in the bladder pressures was noted in the majority of patients. At present, botulinum toxin is being used by some for those individuals with OAB from non-neurologic causes that are refractory (that is, resistant to treatment) to all other medical therapies but without FDA approval for any indication related to lower urinary tract dysfunction.

70. What are the possible side effects of the botulinum toxin?

Injections with botulinum toxin are usually well tolerated. Once injected, the toxin diffuses into the surrounding muscle and bladder tissue but its effect decreases with increasing distance from the injection site. If the injection goes beyond the bladder wall, then there may be an effect on muscles and tissue outside of the bladder.

Rarely, the injection of the toxin will be followed by flu-like symptoms. Weakness has been reported, although almost exclusively in non-urologic use. Botulinum toxin should not be used in a pregnant woman or a woman who is breast-feeding. The effects of botulinum toxin in children are not well known. The **cystoscopy** itself and injections may cause a temporary irritation to the urethra and bladder, leading to short-term discomfort with urination (dysuria) and blood in the urine (hematuria). Rarely, an individual can develop a urinary tract infection or urinary retention. Sometimes, though, urinary retention is the goal (such as in the patient on self intermittent catheterization who wets between catheterizations because of involuntary bladder contractions). The long-term effects of botulinum toxin on the bladder muscle are not well known, but there appears to be no scarring produced in the bladder wall.

Cystoscopy

A procedure in which the bladder and urethra are examined through a narrow telescope-like device that is passed through the urethra into the bladder.

71. What is neuromodulation/sacral nerve stimulation?

Neuromodulation, using the Interstim Continence Control System device (Medtronic, Inc., Minneapolis,

MN), is a form of electrical stimulation that was approved by the FDA in 1997 and is in common use all over the world. The technique involves the surgical placement of a permanent continuous nerve stimulator and its electrode wires (see **Figure 14**). The electrode wires are hooked around select "sacral nerve roots," the nerves going to and from the bladder and other pelvic organs, as they exit from the spinal cord.

The mechanism by which sacral nerve stimulation affects bladder dysfunction is not entirely understood. One theory is that urgency and urgency incontinence may be associated with dysfunction of the pelvic floor muscles and the urethral sphincter muscles. It is thought that stimulation of the sacral nerve roots will decrease the "spastic" activity of the pelvic floor muscles and increase the tone of the urethral sphincter. Another possibility is that stimulation of certain nerves, especially sensory nerves in the pelvis, may lead to an inhibition of the nerves that stimulate the bladder to contract.

72. Who is a candidate for sacral neuromodulation?

Candidates for sacral neuromodulation are those individuals who have failed first-line therapies, including behavioral therapy and oral therapy. Sacral neuromodulation may be considered before more invasive surgical procedures such as bladder augmentation and urinary diversion.

All individuals considering sacral neuromodulation should undergo a complete urologic and neurologic evaluation. This evaluation should include: a history; physical examination; urinalysis; radiologic evaluation of the

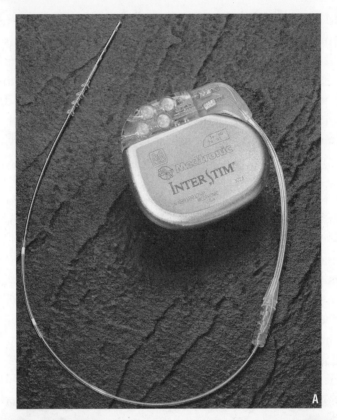

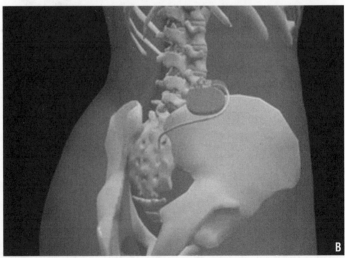

Figure 14   Neuromodulation device. A) Neurostim device. B) Placement of the Neurostim device.

Reprinted with permission from Medtronic, Inc. © 2004.

kidneys, bladder, and lower spinal column including the **sacrum**; a urodynamic study; and a cystoscopy. This extensive evaluation is to ensure that there are no other conditions present that may cause or mimic the OAB symptoms, such as bladder cancer, urinary tract infections, etc.

Sacrum

Refers to the large, irregular, triangular shaped bone made up of the five fused vertebrae below the lumbar region; comprises part of the pelvis.

73. *How is sacral neuromodulation performed?*

There are three stages to the implantation of the Interstim device.

- Phase 1: To identify the proper location of the sacral nerves
- Phase 2: Placement of external wires to test the individual's response to the electrical stimulation
- Phase 3: Implantation of the Interstim device (see Figure 15, Question 71)

Phase 1

This phase may be performed with the patient under local or general anesthesia. The patient is placed in a prone (lying facedown) position. The sacrum is palpated to feel for the openings (foramina) in the sacrum from which the nerve roots emerge. Two needle electrodes, one on each side, are placed into the sacral foramina. Stimulating the electrodes and evaluating the response confirm the proper positioning of the electrodes. If the electrodes are in the proper position, the pelvic floor muscles will contract with stimulation of the needle electrode and the big toe will bend. If the needle electrodes are not in the correct position, they are repositioned until they are in the proper place.

Treatment of Overactive Bladder

Phase 1 may be combined with Phase 2 in the same procedure.

Phase 2

Once the correct position of the needle electrodes is confirmed, external stimulation wires are attached to them. The wires may be taped in place or tunneled under the skin to prevent them from falling out over the following 3- to 4-day test period. The external wires are connected to a portable hand-held neurostimulator. The patient is discharged to home the same day and is asked to complete a **micturition** (voiding) diary over the following 3 to 4 days. A urodynamic study is obtained prior to the fourth day to assess the patient's response. A positive response is an improvement in clinical symptoms by at least 50%. At the end of the 3 to 4 days the wires are removed.

Micturition

The act of voiding urine or urination.

Phase 3

Those patients who responded positively during the trial with the external stimulation wires are candidates for implantation of the permanent device. Typically, there is at least a 2-week interval between removal of the external stimulation wires and placement of the permanent device, to decrease the chance of developing an infection. This procedure is performed under general anesthesia. One or, more commonly, two (one on each side) permanent electrodes are placed into the sacral canal via the third sacral foramina in the pelvis. To prevent movement of the electrode it is secured in place. The wires are tunneled under the skin to bring them to the stimulating device, which is placed under the skin in the groin or buttock area.

74. What is the success rate of sacral neuromodulation?

Of those individuals with refractory (resistant to treatment) urgency incontinence, approximately 50 to 60% will have a positive response to the test stimulation. In those who have a positive response with test stimulation and who undergo permanent implantation, there is a durable positive result for at least 5 years in about 60% of the individuals.

Studies in women with an average age between 43 and 50 years demonstrated that about 40% of the women remained dry over the long term and the remainder noted a more than 50% improvement in their urge incontinent episodes. A study of 25 patients older than 55 years of age with refractory urge incontinence demonstrated that 25 (48%) had a positive response to the test stimulation. After implantation of the permanent device, all 25 noted a more than 50% reduction in their urge incontinent episodes and two individuals became totally dry.

In another study, 51 patients with refractory urgency incontinence and a positive response to Phase 2 were randomized to either a control group or a stimulation group. Compared to the control group, the stimulation group demonstrated statistically significant improvements with respect to the number of voids daily, volume voided, and the degree of urgency. In addition, the stimulation group demonstrated statistically significant improvements in quality of life when compared to the control group. Remember all of these patients enrolled in these studies were refractory to the standard pharmacologic and behavioral therapy.

Individuals who do not tend to respond as well to Interstim include male patients with refractory urgency incontinence and those individuals whose first involuntary bladder contraction occurs at a small bladder volume. The latter underscores the need for urodynamic studies prior to performing the procedure. Lastly, individuals with significant psychological or psychiatric problems with OAB tend to fail therapy more often that individuals without psychological problems for unknown reasons.

75. What are the risks of placement of a sacral neuromodulation device?

Overall, the complication rate is 22% to 43% with a re-operation rate of 6% to 33%. Complications may be related to the surgical procedure or to the function of the device.

Surgical related complications include:

- Discomfort related to placement and tunneling of the electrode wires and the neurostimulator device
- Wound infections and infections around the neurostimulator device
- Migration of the electrodes

Complications related to the device itself include:

- Uncomfortable sensations related to too high of an electrical current
- Broken electrodes
- Mechanical problems with the device
- Battery exhaustion

76. Are there other forms of electrical stimulation besides sacral nerve stimulation?

Yes, there are other forms of electrical stimulation that have been used to treat a variety of voiding troubles. Pelvic floor electrostimulation has been used to strengthen the sphincter, the muscles around the urethra, and the pelvic floor muscles. These forms of stimulation may be **transcutaneous** by placing the stimulator device on the skin in the appropriate area. Other nerves have been used, such as the pudendal nerve (also in the pelvis) and the posterior tibial nerve (in the lower leg). Studies on the results of stimulation of these two sites are ongoing.

Transcutaneous

Denotes the passage of substances through the unbroken skin.

77. What is bladder augmentation?

Bladder augmentation is a surgical procedure whereby the bladder is enlarged. The increase in size may be by the addition of other tissues, such as a segment of intestine, a segment of the stomach, or utilization of a segment of dilated ureter (see **Figure 15**).

In addition, the bladder may be enlarged functionally by removing the detrusor muscle covering the bladder lining, called the **mucosa**, thus allowing the mucosa in that area to expand. The goals of bladder augmentation are to:

Mucosa

A mucous tissue lining various tubular structures, including the bladder, similar to the lining of the inside of your mouth.

• Enable storage of urine at a low bladder pressure
• Help the patient achieve continence
• Avoid damage to the kidneys
• Allow the patient to empty his/her bladder in a timely and convenient manner

111

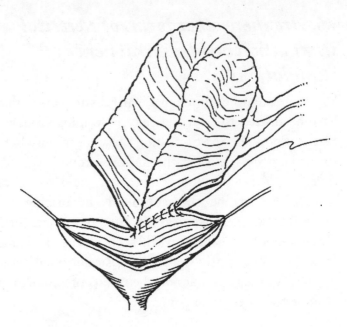

Figure 15 Bladder augmentation

78. Who is a candidate for bladder augmentation?

Bladder augmentation is not considered a first-line therapy for the management of OAB. In fact, it is considered only when all other methods of treatment have failed. Individuals who are undergoing bladder augmentation must be willing to take the risk that they will be dependent on **clean intermittent catheterization (CIC)** to empty their bladder for the rest of their life. Most people can learn how to perform this procedure. First, the patient must learn his or her own urological anatomy. He or she also must be able to reach the urethra and learn how to manipulate the catheter (tube) to empty the bladder properly.

Candidates should also be aware of the permanent nature of the procedure and the risks related to the type of bladder augmentation being performed. Those

Clean intermittent catheterization

A process using a type of temporary catheter to remove urine from the body on a regular basis throughout the day; usually self-accomplished by inserting the tube through the urethra to empty the bladder on a periodic basis.

individuals with small bladder capacities, elevated bladder pressures, and involuntary bladder contractions with normal urethral sphincter function are the best candidates for bladder augmentation.

79. What are the types of bladder augmentation?

There are several different ways to enlarge the bladder including **enterocystoplasty, gastrocystoplasty, autoaugmentation**, and **ureterocystoplasty**. There are studies being performed to determine the feasibility of growing bladder cells in the laboratory to use for bladder augmentation.

Enterocystoplasty

Enterocystoplasty is the most common method for bladder augmentation. It is the procedure to which all other bladder enlargement procedures are compared. With enterocystoplasty, the bladder is made larger by the addition of a segment of small or large intestine. Traditionally, the ileum, which is a segment of the small intestine, is used. The piece of intestine is isolated from the remainder of the intestine and the continuity of the remaining intestine re-established. The isolated piece of intestine is then opened and reconfigured as a patch (see Figure 15). It is important that the intestinal piece is opened and reconfigured, since leaving it in its normal shape as a tube would be like sewing a windsock onto the bladder. This would not increase the holding capacity by much. The surgery is performed under general anesthesia. Typically it is performed through a midline abdominal cut (**incision**); however, some **urologists** are performing all or part of

Enterocystoplasty

A surgical procedure to enlarge the bladder by the addition of a segment of small or large intestine.

Gastrocystoplasty

Similar to enterocystoplasty, except that instead of using a piece of intestine, a segment of the stomach is used to patch the bladder.

Autoaugmentation

A surgical procedure in which a part of the bladder muscle is removed from the underlying mucosa, allowing it to expand.

Ureterocystoplasty

Technique is used in patients who have a dilated distal ureter, which can be isolated, opened, and used as a bladder patch.

Incision

A cut, a surgical wound.

Urologist

A physician who has completed a medical degree as well as advanced training and practice in the field of urology; is concerned with the study, diagnosis, and treatment of the genitourinary tract.

Treatment of Overactive Bladder

Laparoscopically

A type of micro-surgery using a tiny laparoscope passed through the skin and into the organ, with a fiber-optic camera and surgical tools inserted to view and perform the surgery.

Cystogram

A type of test where fluid called contrast material is inserted through a catheter placed into the bladder and X-rays are obtained. The contrast material causes specific areas of the body to be "lit up" by the X-rays, so that the radiologist can analyze the area.

the procedure **laparoscopically**. It is important that the bladder be opened fully, as this helps prevent involuntary bladder contractions and increases in bladder pressure after the procedure. The intestinal patch is then sewn to the bladder. Typically, a drainage tube, called a Foley catheter or a suprapubic tube, is left in place for at least 1 week to allow for healing. The hospital stay is usually around 5 to 7 days, depending on when bowel function returns. A **cystogram**, a study in which contrast material is inserted through the drainage tube into the bladder and X-rays obtained, is performed to rule out any leaks prior to the tube removal.

Advantages of enterocystoplasty include:

- The presence of adequate amounts of intestine in most individuals
- Long-term success rates; up to 77% of patients with intractable OAB are dry with ileal enterocystoplasty
- Increases in bladder capacity

Disadvantages of enterocystoplasty include:

- Early complications related to enterocystoplasty include: bleeding, infection, urinary leakage, and wound breakdown.
- Late complications related to enterocystoplasty include: intra-abdominal adhesions leading to a bowel obstruction, urinary tract infections, bladder and kidney stones, and bladder rupture.
- Production of mucus by the bowel segment may require bladder irrigation to prevent obstruction, infections, and stone formation.
- Long-term risk of malignancy; this is rare and in the few patients who developed a cancer, it was

identified 15 years or more after the augmentation. Because of this risk it is recommended that periodic surveillance with a cystoscopy (look into the bladder with a telescope) and a **urine cytology** (examination of the urine for abnormal cells) be performed. To perform a urine cytology, a small amount of urine is sent to a pathologist, who examines it to determine the presence or absence of any cancer cells in the urine.

Urine cytology
A small amount of urine is sent to the pathologist, who examines the urine sample to determine the presence or absence of any cancer cells.

- Although some individuals may be able to void spontaneously after bladder augmentation, all patients must be prepared to perform lifelong clean intermittent catheterization.

- Electrolyte abnormalities may occur with enterocystoplasty. The isolated segment of intestine continues to function like a normal intestine. It is able to absorb certain chemicals in the urine. Because of this absorption of chemicals from the urine, periodic blood testing is required. Some individuals will require the addition of medications to counteract the acid that is reabsorbed by the intestinal segment.

Autoaugmentation

Autoaugmentation is the surgical procedure in which a part of the bladder muscle—the detrusor—is removed from the bladder. By removing the detrusor from a segment of the bladder, the ability of that segment to contract is destroyed, and the mucosa (lining) pouches out, increasing the bladder capacity. Since the procedure requires access only to the bladder, the surgery does not require entry into the abdominal cavity, only the pelvis.

Advantages of autoaugmentation include:

- Less invasive procedure than enterocystoplasty
- No risk of bowel obstruction

- Faster recovery than enterocystoplasty
- Effective in decreasing uninhibited bladder contractions

Disadvantages of autoaugmentation include:

- Lack of consistent improvement in bladder capacity; consequently it is not often used
- May require clean intermittent catheterization for bladder emptying

Ureterocystoplasty

Ureterocystoplasty is a technique used in patients who have a dilated distal ureter which can be isolated, opened, and used as a bladder patch.

Advantages of ureterocystoplasty include:

- Use of native urothelial tissue, which behaves like the normal tissue lining the bladder and, thus, there is no mucus production.
- Does not require entry into the abdominal cavity and, thus, there is no risk of a bowel obstruction or bowel adhesions.

Disadvantages of ureterocystoplasty include:

Vesicoureteral reflux

Urine passing backward from the bladder to the kidney.

- It cannot be used in most patients because it requires that the individual have a greatly dilated ureter, which is not common. Candidates for this procedure are those with high-grade **vesicoureteral reflux** (urine passing backwards from the bladder to the kidney) or those with an obstructed distal ureter. Typically, this procedure is performed in infants who are born with structural abnormalities that cause the ureter to dilate.

- Requires either removal of the ipsilateral kidney or a simultaneous procedure to establish drainage of the kidney. When the distal ureter is separated from the proximal ureter, the proximal ureter needs to be reconnected to the bladder or to the ureter on the opposite side of the body; this permits the urine from the kidney to drain out of the kidney and into the bladder. If this cannot be done or the kidney is not functioning, then the kidney needs to be removed.

- Although it appears that those individuals who are voiding on their own and who undergo ureterocystoplasty have a greater likelihood of being able to void on their own after the surgery, there is still the chance that the bladder will not empty adequately. That would require long-term, clean intermittent catheterization for bladder emptying.

Other Techniques Being Investigated

Animal studies have shown that it is possible to make the ureter dilate over time, and when the ureter is adequately dilated, a ureterocystoplasty can be performed. This procedure has not been done yet in humans, however. It would carry the same advantages of a straightforward ureterocystoplasty, but would require additional time and an additional procedure to dilate the normal ureter.

Since many of the problems related to enterocystoplasty are due to the ability of the lining of the intestine to release (secrete) and take up (reabsorb) chemicals in the urine, basic scientists and urologists have looked at whether just the lining of the intestine could be removed and used as a patch. This preliminary technique has been used in a few humans, but the numbers of patients who have undergone this procedure are too small to make any strong conclusions and long-term information is limited.

Tissue engineering

A pioneering technique of growing cells designed to mimic the behavior and keep reproducibility of normal cells.

Research currently is focused on **tissue engineering** of bladders using cell transplantation. This is an exciting area of research, since theoretically it would allow a few cells from an individual's bladder to be removed and grown in the proper laboratory setting in sheets, so that the different layers of the bladder develop. These sheets of cells could then be transplanted directly into the bladder. This might be the ideal technique for bladder augmentation, but it is still in the experimental stages and will require much more testing before it can be used in humans.

80. What are bladder denervation procedures?

Bladder denervation procedures are designed to interrupt the nerve supply to the bladder. By interrupting the nerves that stimulate the bladder muscle to contract, it can prevent bladder contractions. If the sensory fibers in the bladder are interrupted, then this may also prevent bladder contractions and urgency because it prevents the bladder from sending messages to the central nervous system. Since neurologic control of bladder function occurs centrally (in the brain and spinal column), peripherally, and within the bladder itself, new techniques have focused on interrupting cell signaling in these areas. These procedures may be reversible or irreversible (permanent).

Reversible Procedures

The simplest form of bladder denervation is **mucosal anesthesia**. An anesthetic agent is placed into the urethra, bladder, or rectum. This will only affect the sensory fibers. In theory, if the patient responds to this procedure, it would confirm that the problem is one of bladder sensation stimulating the over activity.

Local anesthesia can be injected into the sacrum to block the sacral nerves supplying the bladder. Alternatively a spinal anesthetic can be administered.

Irreversible Procedures

In individuals with an OAB secondary to spinal cord injury, specialized spinal surgery to interrupt the nerves stimulating the bladder has been effective. However, after this procedure the bladder fails to contract, and the patient must empty his/her bladder by clean intermittent catheterization.

In females with refractory OAB, a transvaginal procedure called the **Ingelman-Sundberg procedure** has been used by some. Prior to surgery the nerves that would be denervated by the procedure (between the vagina and the bladder) are injected with a local anesthetic. If the woman notes an improvement in her symptoms, then the procedure is carried out. This procedure is not used often, and thus results on only a small number of patients are available.

Mucosal anesthesia

A type of procedure still being studied where an anesthetic agent is placed into the urethra, bladder, or rectum, to affect the sensory fibers in the bladder. In theory, if the patient responds to this procedure, it would confirm that the problem is one of bladder sensation stimulating the over activity.

Local anesthesia

A short-acting spinal anesthetic or intravenous sedation.

Ingelman-Sundberg procedure

A transvaginal surgical technique to destroy some of the nerves supplying the bladder to achieve control over involuntary bladder contractions.

Glossary

Acetylcholine: The chemical which is released from the pelvic nerves and causes contraction of the bladder muscle cells by attaching to a specialized component (receptor) on the bladder muscle cell membrane.

Acontractile bladder: A bladder that does not contract.

Afferent pathway: Messages (nerve impulse signals) inflowing to the central nervous system (brain and spinal cord) from the bladder/urethra.

Alpha receptor agonists: Type of medication that causes the muscles around the urethra, the sphincter muscles, to tighten or contract; may also cause tightening of the muscles that surround arteries and thus result in high blood pressure.

Angiocatheter: A small tube inserted into a blood vessel. Dye is injected into it so that the surrounding blood vessels and capillaries can be visualized to determine if there is a leak.

Antimuscarinic: A type of medication that blocks the attachment of the neurotransmitter responsible for normal bladder contraction to the receptor on the bladder muscle cells that initiates the process of contraction when activated by the neurotransmitter acetylcholine. They also may block sensory (afferent) impulses from the bladder back to the central nervous system.

Atrophic vaginitis: Changes in the vaginal lining and wall caused by low or absent estrogen levels before or after menopause or after hysterectomy and oophorectomy.

Autoaugmentation: A surgical procedure in which a part of the bladder muscle is removed from the underlying mucosa, allowing it to expand.

Behaviorial therapy: A group of treatments designed for educating an individual about his/her medical condition and the function of the organ affected so strategies can be developed to minimize or eliminate the symptoms.

Biofeedback: Information about one or more of an individual's normally unconscious body processes is made available to the individual through a visual (see), auditory (hear), or tactile (touch) signal.

Bladder augmentation: A surgical procedure whereby the bladder is enlarged with patches of organ tissue from the colon or a synthetic substance.

Bladder denervation: Techniques to deaden or eliminate the nerves going to the, bladder in an effort to interrupt the nerve supply to the bladder and stop bladder contractions.

Bladder outlet: Area where the bladder joins the urethra.

Blood brain barrier (BBB): Semipermeable network of the tiniest blood vessels called capillaries with special endothelial cells surrounding the brain; the barrier prevents a variety of agents such as medications from passing through and entering the brain. Its function is to protect the brain from potentially harmful substances (like certain medications), other neurotransmitters, and hormones in the body, and to maintain the brain in a constant environment.

Botulinum neurotoxin: One of the most poisonous biologic chemicals known; produced by the bacterium Clostridium botulinum; very small amounts can lead to paralysis. Not approved by the FDA but used to treat OAB by injection of small amounts into multiple areas in the bladder muscle layer.

Capsaicin: The active ingredient found in chili peppers; may be instilled into the bladder to decrease bladder activity. Not FDA approved.

Catheter: A tube usually made of latex or silicone especially designed to be passed through the urethra into the bladder to drain the bladder.

Central nervous system: Found in the brain and spinal cord; responsible for starting or preventing urination.

Clean intermittent catheterization: A process using a type of temporary catheter to remove urine from the body on a regular basis throughout the day; usually self-accomplished by inserting the tube through the urethra to empty the bladder on a periodic basis.

Cognition: General term encompassing thinking, learning, and memory.

Compliance: The consistency and accuracy with which a patient follows the regimen prescribed by a physician or other healthcare professional.

Compliance, bladder: The ability of the bladder to store urine at low pressures.

Congenital anomalies: Existing at birth; refers to physical traits, conditions, diseases, abnormalities, or malformations, etc., which may be either hereditary or the result of an influence occurring during gestation up to the moment of birth.

Continence: Ability to retain urine and/or feces until a proper time for their discharge.

Cystocele: Hernia-like disorder in women that occurs when the wall between the bladder and the vagina weakens and the bladder drops into the vagina.

Cystogram: A type of test where fluid called contrast material is inserted through a catheter placed into the bladder and X-rays are obtained. The contrast material causes specific areas of the body to be "lit up" by the X-rays, so that the radiologist can analyze the area.

Cystometrogram (CMG): Recording of bladder pressure during filling and emptying.

Cystoscope: A long telescope-like instrument that is passed through the urethra into the bladder for diagnostic and therapeutic purposes. It allows one to visualize inside the bladder and urethra.

Cystoscopy: A procedure in which the bladder and urethra are examined through a narrow telescope-like device that is passed through the urethra into the bladder.

Darifenacin (Enablex, Novartis): An antimuscarinic agent that is relatively selective for the M3 receptor, the one responsible for bladder contractility in the normal bladder. No apparent side effects on the brain or heart.

Detrusor: Another name given to the muscle which comprises the bladder contractile mechanism. Coordinated contraction of the detrusor and opening of the bladder outlet allows for normal urination.

Diverticula: Pouch or sac outpouching from a tubular or saccular organ such as the gut or bladder.

Efferent pathway: Messages (nerve impulse signals) outflowing from the central nervous system to the organs (the bladder for example).

Efficacy: Extent to which a specific intervention, procedure, regimen, or service produces a beneficial result under ideal conditions.

Electromyography (EMG): Recording of the electric potential from your pelvic floor muscles (spincter muscles) during bladder filling and emptying.

Enterocele: Occurs when your small intestine (small bowel) drops into the lower pelvic cavity and protrudes into your vagina, creating a bulge. An enterocele is a vaginal hernia.

Enterocystoplasty: A surgical procedure to enlarge the bladder by the addition of a segment of small or large intestine.

Estrogens: A class of drugs, orally or topically applied, which may be used by urologists and urogynecologists to make the urethral tissue healthier.

Fascia: A sheet of connective tissue covering or binding together body structures.

Fesoterodine: The newest antimuscarinic available in 2 once daily doses.

Fluoroscopy: Visualization of tissues and deep structures of the body by X-ray.

Frequency volume chart: A document plotting the amount of urine and number of times an individual urinates over a period of time.

Functional incontinence: A situation in which the bladder, urethra, and pelvic floor muscles are functioning properly, but physical or mental function interferes with one's ability to independently get to the bathroom on time.

Gastrocystoplasty: Similar to enterocystoplasty, except that instead of using a piece of intestine, a segment of the stomach is used to patch the bladder.

Hematoma: A collection of blood that forms in a tissue, organ, or body space as a result of a broken blood vessel.

Hypertension: Transitory or sustained elevated arterial blood pressure. Untreated, it can cause cardiovascular damage.

Imipramine: An antidepressant medication sometimes used for overactive bladder; it has antimuscarinic properties and acts on two neurotransmitters in the brain and spinal cord (serotonin and noradrenaline) involved in the complex interactions related to normal bladder filling and emptying.

Incision: A cut, a surgical wound.

Ingelman-Sundberg procedure: A transvaginal surgical technique to destroy some of the nerves supplying the bladder to achieve control over involuntary bladder contractions.

Intravesical: Medication placed directly into the bladder.

Involuntary bladder contractions: Bladder contractions that occur during the filling/storage phase of bladder function. They may be associated with urinary frequency, urgency, and urgency incontinence.

Kegel exercises: Exercises designed to strengthen weak pelvic floor muscles.

Laparoscopically: A type of microsurgery using a tiny laparoscope passed through the skin and into the abdomen, with a fiber-optic camera and surgical tools inserted to view and perform the surgery.

Local anesthesia: A short-acting spinal anesthetic or intravenous sedation.

Lower urinary tract symptoms (LUTS): Term used to describe storage and emptying symptoms.

Micturition: The act of voiding urine or urination.

Mixed urinary incontinence: Involuntary leakage of urine associated with urgency as well as with exertion, effort, sneezing, or coughing. The combination of urge incontinence and stress urinary incontinence.

Mucosa: A mucous tissue lining various tubular structures, including the bladder, similar to the lining of the inside of your mouth.

Mucosal anesthesia: A type of procedure still being studied where an anesthetic agent is placed into the urethra, bladder, or rectum, to affect the sensory fibers in the bladder. In theory, if the patient responds to this procedure, it would confirm that the problem is one of bladder sensation stimulating the over activity.

Muscarinic receptor: A membrane-bound protein that contains a recognition site for acetylcholine; combination of acetylcholine with the receptor initiates a physiologic change (i.e., slowing of the heart rate, increased glandular activity, and stimulation of smooth muscle contractions).

Neuromodulation: Surgical placement of a permanent continuous nerve stimulator and its electrode wires to alter the function of the organ(s) innervated by that nerve or nerves.

Nocturia: Having to wake from sleep at night to urinate after a day of normal fluid intake; causes include increased urine production at night, incomplete bladder emptying, sleep problems, or overactive bladder.

Obstruction: Outflow of urine from the bladder is blocked; may be caused by prostate enlargement or urethral strictures, narrowed areas in the urethra, or medications that affect the function of the urethra, among others.

Orthostatic hypotension: Lowering of blood pressure while moving from a sitting or supine position to a standing position; potential for dizziness and collapsing.

Overactive bladder: A symptom complex characterized by urgency, with or without urgency urinary incontinence, usually with frequency and nocturia often associated with involuntary contractions of the bladder (detrusor overactivity).

Oxybutynin: One of the oldest pharmaceutical therapies for overactive bladder. It is effective, but its use is limited by a high incidence of side effects, including dry mouth and constipation.

Oxybutynin extended release (Ditropan XL): A type of pharmaceutical therapy for overactive bladder. It is similar to oxybutynin but is a sustained release formulation with less dry mouth and constipation than immediate release oxybutynin.

Pelvic floor muscles: A series of muscles that form a sling or hammock across the outlet of the pelvis; these muscles, together with their surrounding tissue, are responsible for keeping all of the pelvic organs (bladder, uterus, and rectum) in place and functioning correctly.

Pelvic prolapse: A weakening in the web of muscles at the base of the pelvis causing a protrusion of the bladder, urethra, uterus, or rectum into the vagina and possibly beyond (beyond the vaginal introitus).

Perineum: Area between the thighs extending from the tail bone (coccyx) to the pubis (between the vulva and anus in the female and scrotum and anus in the male) and lying below the pelvic diaphragm.

Peripheral nervous system: Nerves in the body other than in the brain and spinal cord.

Poor contractility: A situation in which the bladder cannot generate and/or sustain a contraction capable of completely emptying it of urine.

Poorly compliant bladder: Holds urine at higher than normal bladder pressures, causing poor emptying of the kidneys, a backup of urine in the kidneys, and eventually kidney damage.

Post-void residual urine: The amount of urine left in the bladder after voiding; if elevated may lead to urinary tract infections, bladder stones, further distention of the bladder, worsening of bladder function, or dilation of the kidneys and ureter.

Potty training: Ability of toddlers to learn how to hold their urine and then voluntarily empty the bladder at a socially acceptable time and in a socially acceptable place.

Propantheline bromide: A nonselective antimuscarinic medication for overactive bladder; individual doses will vary.

Propiverine: An antimuscarinic agent that is used in Europe for the management of overactive bladder. Propiverine is not approved for use in the United States.

Radical prostatectomy: Removal of the entire prostate, a procedure performed for prostate cancer.

Rectocele: Occurs when the fascia—a wall of fibrous tissue separating the rectum from the vagina—becomes weakened, allowing the front wall of the rectum to bulge into the vagina.

Resiniferatoxin: A chemical derived from a cactus-like plant, Euphorbia resinifera, which may be instilled into the bladder to decrease bladder activity.

Sacrum: Refers to the large, irregular, triangular shaped bone made up of the five fused vertebrae below the lumbar region; comprises part of the pelvis.

Skin patch electrodes: A noninvasive, no-pain method used in testing muscle activity or pressures involving a flat adhesive patch with embedded wires.

Small capacity bladder: Organ cannot hold much urine because of fibrosis or scarring or neurologic causes; the bladder loses its elasticity so the individual must urinate more frequently.

Solifenacin (Vesicare, Astellas): An antimuscarinic agent used in the treatment of overactive bladder.

Sphincter mechanism: The muscular mechanism that helps to maintain continence.

Stasis: A circumstance in which high pressure in the bladder causes a backup of urine within the ureter and eventually the kidney. Stasis of urine may also occur in the bladder if there is decreased bladder contractility or bladder outlet obstruction.

Stress incontinence: Also known as genuine stress urinary incontinence, (GSUI), involuntary loss of bladder control during periods of increased abdominal pressure such as coughing, laughing, heavy lifting, or straining.

Timed or prophylactic voiding: A type of therapy that involves urinating at 2- to 3-hour intervals, no matter if there is an urge to void or not.

Tissue engineering: A pioneering technique of growing cells designed to mimic the behavior and reproducibility of normal cells.

Tolterodine (Detrol): First antimuscarinic drug developed solely for use in overactive bladder.

Tolterodine, (Detrol LA): Type of antimuscarinic drug developed in a capsule containing small micropheres that are released slowly into the body, allowing for a sustained release of medication; used for overactive bladder and has a lower incidence of side effects.

Transcutaneous: Denotes the passage of substances through the unbroken skin.

Transdermal: Medication is delivered to the body by a skin patch or a gel.

Transdermal oxybutynin (Oxytrol): A patch formulation of oxybutynin that is changed twice a week. The patch delivers 3.9mg of oxybutynin per day.

Transdermal oxybutynin gel (Gelnique): A gel formulation of oxybutynin that is applied to select areas of the skin once daily and is associated with a lower incidence of side effects than other formulations of oxybutynin.

Transient (temporary) incontinence: Leakage of urine caused by illness or medications that temporarily cause functional incontinence.

Transurethral prostatectomy (TURP): Removal of the central portion of the prostate to make the outlet wider and reduce obstruction.

Transurethral resection: Removal of the center portion of the prostate to make the outlet wider and reduce obstruction.

Tricyclic antidepressants: A class of medications which may be used to treat incontinence. They lower the bladder pressure by relaxing the bladder muscle and also help further by tightening the sphincter muscle.

Trospium chloride (Sanctura, Sanctura XR): An antimuscarinic medication that is approved for the treatment of overactive bladder; it is unlikely to penetrate the brain and thus does not appear to affect cognitive function.

Ultrasound: A noninvasive test using radio waves (frequency greater than 30,000 MHz); used to evaluate the kidneys and bladder to assess bladder emptying capacity.

Ureter: A long, thin, hollow tubular structure connecting the kidneys to the bladder. The ureter propels urine from the kidneys into the bladder.

Ureterocystoplasty: Technique is used in patients who have a dilated distal ureter, which can be isolated, opened, and used as a bladder patch.

Urethra: Canal leading from the bladder to the body's skin to discharge urine externally. In the female, it is ~4cm long and opens in the perineum between the clitoris and vaginal opening; in the male it is ~20cm long and opens in the glans penis.

Urethral sphincter: A muscle that closes the urethra when contracted.

Urge (urgency) incontinence: Unintended leakage or loss of urine into clothing associated with urgency.

Urinalysis: A type of test of the urine to determine normalcy or abnormality.

Urinary frequency: Having to void more than eight times per day with normal intake of fluids.

Urinary incontinence: Involuntary loss of urine. May be the result of an overactive bladder, stress incontinence, functional incontinence, or other causes.

Urinary retention, acute: The inability to urinate on one's own.

Urinary urgency: Sudden compelling desire to urinate that often is difficult to defer.

Urinate: To excrete urine.

Urine cytology: A small amount of urine is sent to the pathologist, who examines the urine sample to determine the presence or absence of any cancer cells.

Urodynamic study: A test which evaluates the ability of the bladder to fill with and store urine as well as to empty; the function of the outlet is to remain closed during bladder filling and to stay open during bladder emptying; study determines the presence or absence of outlet obstruction.

Uroflow: The rate of flow of the urine stream; often a component of a urodynamic study, but may be performed in the office.

Urogynecologist: A specialty trained physician who has completed a medical degree as well as advanced train-ing and practice in the fields of Ob/Gyn; is concerned with the study, diagnosis, and treatment of the genitourinary tract and gynecology as well as the study, diagnosis, and treatment of the female genital tract, endocrinology, and the reproductive physiology of the female.

Urologist: A physician who has completed a medical degree as well as advanced training and practice in the field of urology; is concerned with the study, diagnosis, and treatment of the genitourinary tract in the male and the urinary tract in the female.

Urothelium: The innermost lining layer of the urinary tract.

Vesicoureteral reflux: Urine passing backward from the bladder to the kidney.

Video-urodynamics: Use of intermittent fluoroscopy (taking X-rays) during the urodynamic study to visualize the bladder and urethra.

Void: To evacuate urine.

Warning time: Duration of time between the individual's initial perception of urinary urgency and the onset of voiding or leakage.

Index

Italicized page numbers indicate a figure/table. Tables are noted with a *t.*

A

Acetylcholine, 6
  antimuscarinics and blocking of, 67
  botulinum and, 101
  muscarinic receptors and, *68*
Acidic foods, bladder irritation and, 57, 60
Acontractile bladder, 10
Additive effects, 92
A delta fiber, in bladder, 97
Afferent pathway, 24, 25, 67, 69
Age
  nocturia and, 35
  overactive bladder and, 24
  prevalence of overactive bladder by, *27*
Alcohol-based drinks, restricting, nocturia
    management and, 39
Alfuzosin (Uroxatral), 35, 55
Alpha-adrenergic receptor blockers, 54
Alpha blockers, prostatic enlargement
    and, 35
Alzheimer's disease, overactive bladder and,
    26
Anticholinergics
  additive effects with, 92
  available forms of, 69–70
  prostatic enlargement and, 35
Antidepressants, 77–78
Antimuscarinic medications, 52, 73, 74, 77
  available forms of, 69–70
  behavioral therapy combined with, 65–66
  constipation and, 88
  contraindications for, 69
  drug-drug interactions with, 92–95
    additive effects, 92
    metabolism-related side effects,
    92–95
  dry mouth and, 91
  efficacy of, 78
  how they work, 67
  side effects of, 81–84

Artificial sweeteners, overactive bladder and,
    57
Astellas, 70
Atrophic vaginitis
  overactive bladder and, 26
  urinary incontinence and, 21
Autoaugmentation, advantages/
    disadvantages with, 114–115
Autonomic dysreflexia, 100
Avodart, 56

B

BBB. *See* Blood brain barrier
Behavioral modification, 31, 33, 61
Behavioral therapy, 52, *52*, 66
  methods within, 56–57
  success rate of, 58–59
Benadryl, 92
Benign enlargement of the prostate gland,
    overactive bladder and, 24, 25
Beta-3 agonists, new, studies of, 95
Beta-3 receptors, in bladder muscle, 95
Bioelectrical signals, 5
Biofeedback, 62, 66
  description of, 64
  location for performance of, 65
  success rate of, 65
Bladder, *4*
  acontractile, 10
  adult, normal capacity of, 2
  defined, 2
  evaluating, 44
  function and anatomy of, 2–7
  malignant conditions of, 21
  pelvic nerve innervation of, *5*
  poor contractility of, 10
Bladder augmentation, 32, 53, 104, *111*
  autoaugmentation, 114–115
  candidates for, 111–112
  description of and goals related to, 110
  enterocystoplasty, 112–114

types of, 112–116
ureterocystoplasty, 115–116
Bladder cancer, 16
Bladder catheter, 47
Bladder compliance, 48
Bladder denervation procedures, 32
  description of, 117
  reversible and irreversible, 118
Bladder diaries, 87
Bladder distention, checking for, 42
Bladder function problems, 8–10
  emptying problems, 9–10
  storage problems, 8–9
Bladder health questionnaires, simplified, 40
Bladder outlet, 4, *4*
  obstruction, 34
    overactive bladder and, 24, 25
Bladder pain syndrome, 15
Bladder stones, 21, 26
Blood brain barrier, 82
Botulinum neurotoxin, 53
  description of, 100
  effectiveness of, in OAB, 102
  overactive bladder and, 101
  side effects with, 103
Botulinum toxin type A (Botox), 49, 66, 100
  how it works, *102*
  investigational studies on, 31, 32
Bowel, muscarinic receptors in, 81, *81*
Bowel regimen, 89–90
BPH. *See* Benign enlargement of the
    prostate gland
Brain, muscarinic receptors in, 81, *81*
Breast-feeding, botulinum toxin contra-
    indication and, 103

C

Caffeine, as diuretic, 57, 60
Capsaicin, 96–97
  effectiveness of, 98–99
  function of, 97–98
  side effects of, 99–100
Cardiovascular disease, 35
Cardura, 35, 55
Casopitant, 95
Central nervous system, 4, 82
Cerebrovascular accident, overactive bladder
    and, 24, 26
C fibers, in bladder, 97
Childbirth, pelvic floor muscles and, 61
Children, overactive bladder in, 28
CIC. *See* Clean intermittent catheterization
Citrucel, 89

Clean intermittent catheterization, 111
Clinical trials, for new OAB medications,
    95–96
Clostridium botulinum, 100
CMG. *See* Cystometrogram
Cognition, antimuscuranics and, 81
Colace, 89
Colon, muscarinic receptors in, 82
Compliance, 58
Congenital anomalies, 10
Congestive heart failure, nocturia and, 38
Constipation, 73
  antimuscuranics and, 81, 82
  defined, 87–88
Continence, 4
CVA. *See* Cerebrovascular accident
CYP3A4 inhibitors, 94
Cystocele, 33
Cystogram, 113
Cystometrogram, 48
Cystoscope, 44, 101
Cystoscopy, 16, 44, 103, 106
Cytochrome P450 systems
  dosing recommendations and, 93–95
  drug metabolism and, 92
Cytology, 45

D

Darifenacin (Enablex), 35, 53, 69, 76
  dosing, half-life and metabolism rate of,
    80*t*
  dosing recommendations for, 93–94
  side effects with, 86*t*
Daytime urinary frequency, nighttime
    urinary frequency *vs.*, 36–38
DDAVP. *See* Desmopressin
Dementia, overactive bladder and, 26
Desmopressin, sodium levels and,
    39–40
Detrol, 35, 73–74
Detrol IR, 70
Detrol LA, 70, 74, 79
  dosing recommendations for, 94
  side effects with, 86*t*
Detrusor
  bladder stretching and, 2
  removal of, 114
Detrusor overactivity, 18, 24, 66
Diabetes
  evaluating for, 43
  overactive bladder and, 26
Diabetes insipidus, 36, 38
Diabetes mellitus, 35, 38

Diagnosis of overactive bladder
    additional studies, 43–44
    hematuria and, 44–45
    history and physical examination, 42
    initial evaluation, 40
    screening tools, 45
    symptom assessment, 41
    urinalysis, 42–43
    urodynamic tests, 45–50
DIAPPERS acronym, for treatable causes
        of urinary incontinence, 21
Diet, overactive bladder and, 24, 57
Diphenhydramine (Benadryl), 92
Ditropan, 35, 69, 70
Ditropan XL, 70, 71–72
Diuretics ("water pills")
    nocturia and, 37, 39
    urinary frequency and, 8
DO. See Detrusor overactivity
Docusate, 89
Domestic quality of life, overactive bladder
        and, 30
Dosing
    with antimuscarinics, 83–84
    medications for overactive bladder and,
        80t
Double-blind study, 85
Doxazosin (Cardura), 35, 55
Drug-drug interactions, 92–95
Dry mouth (xerostomia), 73
    antimuscuranics and, 81–82
    common causes of, 90–91
    oxybutynin and, 70
    prevalence of, 90
    treatment of, 91
Dutasteride (avodart), 56
Dysfunctional voiding, overactive bladder
        and, 24, 25
Dyspareunia, 1

E
Economic burden, of urge incontinence,
        30–31
EEGs. See Electroencephalographs
Efferent pathway, 25
Efficacy, of pelvic floor muscle exercises,
        63
Ejaculatory dysfunction, alpha-adrenergic
        receptors and, 54, 55
Electrical stimulation, other forms of, 110
Electroencephalographs, 73
Electromyelogram, 49
Electromyography, 47, 64

EMG. See Electromyelogram;
        Electromyography
Emollient laxatives/stool softeners, 89
Employment, overactive bladder and, 30
Emptying/voiding symptoms, 9–10
    enlarged prostate and, 34
    LUTS and, 53, 54
Enablex, 35, 69, 76
    dosing, half-life and metabolism rate of,
        80t
    dosing recommendations for, 93–94
    side effects with, 86t
Enterocystoplasty, 116
Enterocystosplasty
    advantages/disadvantages with, 113–114
    description of, 112
Erectile dysfunction, 5 alpha-reductase
        inhibitors and, 55
Estrogen deficiency, overactive bladder and,
        26
Euphorbia resinifera, 97
Exercise, bowel function regulation and, 89

F
Falls, urinary incontinence and, 30
Fatigue, nocturia and, 30
FDA. See Food and Drug Administration
Females. See also Women
    interstitial cystitis in, 15
    overactive bladder and associated condi-
        tions in, 25
Fesoterodine (Toviaz), 35, 53, 70, 77
    dosing, half-life and metabolism rate of,
        80t
    dosing recommendations for, 94
    side effects with, 86t
Fibercon, 89
Fiber intake, constipation reduction and, 89
Finasteride (proscar), 56
5-alpha-reductase inhibitors, 54, 55–56
Flomax, 35, 55
Fluid intake
    constipation reduction and, 89
    nocturia and, 38, 39
    overactive bladder and, 57, 60
    physical examination and, 42
Fluoroscopy, 47
Foley catheter, 100, 113
Food and Drug Administration, 66
Frequency
    delayed voiding and, 61
    urodynamic study and assessment of, 45
Frequency volume chart, 36

Functional incontinence, 11–12
Furosemide (Lasix), 39

G

Gastrocolic reflex, 89
Gender, OAB treatment and, 53–56. *See also* Females; Males; Men; Women
Glomerulations, 16
Glucose check, 43
GU tract, anatomy of, *3*

H

Half-life, of medications for overactive bladder, 80*t*
Heart, muscarinic receptors in, 81, *81*
Hematuria, evaluation related to, 44–45
Heredity, overactive bladder and, 28–29
Hesitancy, urodynamic study and assessment of, 45
History and physical examination, 42
Hunner's ulcers, 16
Hydrochlorothiazide (HydroDiuril, Microzide), 39
Hydrodistention, 16
HydroDiuril, 39
Hypertension, 100
Hypogastric nerve, 5
Hytrin, 35, 55

I

Imipramine (Tofranil), 77–78, 92
Incision, 112
Incomplete bladder emptying, urodynamic study and assessment of, 46
Incontinence
behavioral therapy and, 58
overactive bladder-related *vs.* stress incontinence, 12–13
urodynamic study and assessment of, 50
Incontinent females, physical examination of, 12–13
Indevus, 70
Inducers, of liver enzymes, 93
Infections, urodynamic study and assessment of, 46
Ingelman-Sundberg procedure, 118
Inhibitor drugs, classification of, 93
Intercourse, interstitial cystitis and pain with, 16
Interstim Continence Control System, 103–104
Interstim device, implantation phases for, 106–107

Interstitial cystitis, 15–16, 26
Involuntary bladder contractions, 66

K

Kegel, Arnold, 61
Kegel exercises
biofeedback and, 65
candidates for, 63–64
description of, 61–63
success with, 63
Kidneys, evaluating, 44
KUC-7483, 95

L

Lactulose, 90
Laparoscopically, 113
Lasix, 39
Laxatives, 89–90
Leakage, 8, 41
chronic retention and, 12
overactive bladder with/without, 20
urgency and, 9
Liver
antimuscarinic drugs metabolized in, 93
drug metabolism in, 84
Local anesthesia, 118
Lower urinary tract obstruction, 36
Lower urinary tract symptoms (LUTS)
prostate problems and, 34–35
types of, 53–54

M

Magnesium hydroxide, 89
Males, overactive bladder and associated conditions in, 25. *See also* Men
Malignant conditions of bladder, 21
M2 receptors, 6, 69, 73
M3 receptors, 6, 68–69, 73
Medical therapy, 31, 33, 34, 59
Medications for overactive bladder
antimuscarinics, 52, 66–70
approved for use in United States, 53
approved for use only in Europe, 53
dosing, half-life and metabolism rate for, 80*t*
under investigation for OAB symptoms, 95–96
transdermal delivery of, 67
Medtronic, Inc., 103
Men. *See also* Males
antimuscarinics and, 83
constipation in, 87
Interstim and, 109
OAB treatment in, 53–56

overactive bladder and physical examination for, 42
prevalence of overactive bladder in, 26
prevalence of urinary incontinence in, 11
urodynamic studies in, 50
Menstruation, interstitial cystitis and, 16
Metabolism rate, medications for overactive bladder and, 80t
Metabolism-related side-effects, 92–95
Metamucil, 89
Methylcellulose, 89
Microzide, 39
Micturition, 107
Milk of magnesia, 89
Mixed urinary incontinence, 11, 15, 62
MN-246, 95
MOM. *See* Milk of magnesia
Mucosa, 110
Mucosal anesthesia, 118
Multiple sclerosis, overactive bladder and, 24, 26
Muscarinic receptors, 6
acetylcholine and, *68*
locations of, throughout body, 81, *81*
types of, 68–69

N
National Association for Continence Survey, 58
Nephrologists, 45
Nervous system, parts of, 4–5
Neurogenic cause, of overactive bladder, 24
Neurokinin (NK)-1 receptor antagonists, 95
Neurological conditions, overactive bladder and, 24
Neuromodulation, 49, 66
Neuromodulation/sacral nerve stimulation, description of, 103–104
Neurostim device, placement of, *105*
Nocturia, 7
defined, 19, 35
fatigue and, 30
managing, 38–40
prostatic enlargement and, 34
Nocturnal polyuria, 36
Noradrenaline, 78
Novartis, 69
Nursing home admissions, urinary incontinence and, 30

O
OAB. *See* Overactive bladder
OAB Awareness Tool, *46*

"OAB dry," gender and, 20, 26
OAB-V8, 45
"OAB wet," gender and, 26
Obesity
pelvic floor muscles and, 61
sleep apnea and, 38
Occupational quality of life, overactive bladder and, 30
Oral magnesium citrate, 90
Orthostatic hypotension, 78
Osmotic laxatives, 89
Overactive bladder, 8, 16. *See also* Diagnosis of overactive bladder; Medications for overactive bladder; Treatment options for overactive bladder
causes of, 24–24
in children, 28
conditions producing symptoms typical of, 21, 25–26
curability of, 33–34
defined, 19
description of, 18–19
diagnosis of, 40
healthcare providers in treatment of, 32–33
heredity and, 28–29
impact of, 29–31
management of, 31–32
natural history of, 27
nocturia and, 35–36
pathophysiology of, *18*
prevalence of, 26
by age, *27*
risk for development of, 28
stress incontinence co-occurring with, *14*, 14–15
symptoms of, 9, 13t
treatability of, 31
with/without urinary incontinence, 20
Oxybutynin (Ditropan), 35, 53, 70–71. *See also* Transdermal oxybutynin
administration of, 71
dosing, half-life and metabolism rate for, 80t
dry mouth with, 70, 71
topical form of (under investigation), 95
Oxybutynin immediate release, 69
Oxybutynin XL, 70
Oxytrol, 70, 79

P
Painful bladder syndrome, 15
Painful urination, urodynamic study and assessment of, 46

Parkinson's disease, overactive bladder and, 24, 26
Peak drug levels, antimuscarinics and, 83–84
Pelvic floor
    electrostimulation of, 110
    muscles of
        description of exercises for, 61–63
        urgency incontinence and, 56
    strengthening exercises for, 58
Pelvic nerve, 5
Pelvic prolapse
    assessing, 42
    overactive bladder and, 21
Pelvic surgery, pelvic floor muscles and, 61
Pepper strengths, in heat units, 97
Perineum, physical examination of, 12, 42
Peripheral nervous system, 4
Phase I trials, for new OAB medications, 95, 96
Phase II trials, for new OAB medications, 95, 96
Phase III trials, for new OAB medications, 96
Phase IV trials, for new OAB medications, 96
Phospha-Soda, 90
Physical examination, 42
Physical quality of life, overactive bladder and, 30
Placebo effects, 87
Placebo response, defined, 85
Placebos, 85
Polycarbonil, 89
Polyethylene glycol, 90
Polyuria, 36
Poor contractility, 10
Poorly compliant bladder, 9
"Poor metabolizers," 93
Post-void dribbling, 34
Post-void Residual, 43, 47
Pregnant women, botulinum toxin contra-indication for, 103
Pressure flow study, 49
prn ("as-needed" basis), 72
Propantheline bromide, 70, 77
Prophylactic (or timed) voiding, 56, 60–61
Propiverine, 53, 70, 76–77
Proscar, 56
Prostate cancer
    overactive bladder and, 24, 25
    ruling out, 42
Prostate examination, 42
Prostate problems
    inflammation/infection, 16

lower urinary tract symptoms and, 34–35
Prostate specific antigen (PSA), 5 alpha-reductase inhibitors and, 55
Psychological quality of life, overactive bladder and, 30
Psyllium, 89
Pudendal nerve, 6
PVR. See Post-void Residual

Q
Quality of life, overactive bladder and, 29–31

R
Radical prostectomy, stress incontinence and, 13
Rectal catheter, 47
Rectal examination, 42
Red blood cells, in urine (hemturia), 44–45
Refractory urgency incontinence, sacral neuromodulation and, 108
Resiniferatoxin (RTX), 31, 32, 53, 96–97
    effectiveness of, 98–99
    function of, 97–98
    side effects of, 99–100
Rome II system, constipation and, 88
RTX. See Resiniferatoxin

S
Sacral nerve stimulation, description of, 103–104
Sacral neuromodulation, 32, 53
    candidates for, 104, 106
    stages in, 106–107
    success rate of, 108–109
Sacral neuromodulation devices, risks with placement of, 109
Sacrum, 106
Saliva production, antimuscuranics and, 81–82
Salivary glands, muscarinic receptors in, 81, 81
Sanctura, 35, 70, 74, 79, 94–95
    dosing, half-life and metabolism rate of, 80t
    side effects with, 86t
Sanctura XR, 70, 75, 79, 94–95
    dosing, half-life and metabolism rate of, 80t
    side effects with, 86t
Scovill scale, 97
Second-line therapies, 53
Serotonin, 78
Sexual quality of life, overactive bladder and, 30

Side effects
of antimuscuranics, 81–84
of botulinum neurotoxin, 103
of capsaicin and resiniferatoxin, 99–100
with OAB medications, 85, 86*t*
Sleep apnea, 36, 37–38
Sleep disorders, 36
Small capacity bladder, 8
Social quality of life, overactive bladder and, 30
Sodium biphosphate, 90
Solifenacin (Vesicare), 35, 53, 70, 75–76
dosing, half-life and metabolism rate of, 80*t*
dosing recommendations for, 94
side effects with, 86*t*
Sorbitol, 90
Specialists, for overactive bladder, 32–33
Spinal cord injury, overactive bladder and, 24, 26
SSR 240600, 95
Stasis, 3
Stones (bladder), ruling out presence of, 44
Stool softeners, 89
Storage/filling symptoms, LUTS and, 53, 54
Storage problems, 8–9
Stress urinary incontinence, 11, 20, 21
impact of, 29
kegel exercises and, 61
overactive bladder and, 26
overactive bladder co-occurring with, *14,* 14–15
physical examination and, 42
symptoms of, 13*t*
Strictures, in ureters and urethra, ruling out, 43, 44
Stroke, overactive bladder and, 24, 26
Symptom assessment, 41

T
TA-5538, 95
Tamsulosin (Flomax), 35, 55
Terazosin (Hytrin), 35, 55
Testosterone, 5 alpha-reductase inhibitors and, 55
Third-line therapies, 53
Timed (or prophylactic) voiding, 56, 60–61
Tissue engineering, 117
Tofranil, 77, 92
Tolterodine (Detrol), 35, 53, 73–74
dosing, half-life and metabolism rate of, 80*t*
dosing recommendations for, 94

Tolterodine immediate release, 70
Tolterodine LA, 70
side effects with, 86*t*
Toviaz, 35, 70
dosing recommendations for, 94
side effects with, 86*t*
Transcutaneous stimulation, 110
Transdermal delivery, of medications, 67
Transdermal oxybutynin, 70, 72–73
dosing, half-life and metabolism rate for, 80*t*
side effects with, 86*t*
Transurethral prostatectomy, stress incontinence and, 13
Treatment options for overactive bladder, 52–118
behavioral modification, 52, *52*
behavioral therapy, 56–57, 58–59
biofeedback, 64–66
bladder augmentation, 110–116
bladder denervation procedures, 117–118
botulinum toxin, 100–103
constipation concerns, 87–90
dietary changes, 57
drug-drug interactions and, 92–95
dry mouth and, 90–91
gender and, 53–56
kegel exercises, 61–64
medications, 66–87, 95–100
neuromodulation/sacral nerve stimulation, 103–109
pharmacologic therapy, 52–53
timed voiding, 60–61
voiding diary, 60
Tricyclic antidepressants, 70
Trospium chloride extended release, 70
approval of, 75
dosing, half-life and metabolism rate of, 80*t*
Trospium chloride (Sanctura), 35, 53, 70, 74–75, 94–95
dosing, half-life and metabolism rate of, 80*t*
side effects with, 86*t*
Trough drug levels, antimuscarinics and, 83–84
Tumors, ruling out presence of, 43, 44

U
Ultrasound, 43
Ureter, 2–3
Ureterocytoplasty, advantages/disadvantages of, 115–116
Ureters, evaluating, 44

Urethra, 4, 44
Urethral sphincter, 4
Urge incontinence, economic burden of,
    30–31
Urgency, 9
    behavioral therapy and, 58
    defined, 19
    measure of, 19–20
    oxybutynin and, 71
    urodynamic study and assessment of, 45
Urgency incontinence, 9
    defined, 19
    delayed voiding and, 61
    pelvic floor muscle exercises and, 62
"Urge to void," urgency vs., 20
Urge urinary incontinence, 9
Urinalysis, 39, 42–43
Urinary bladder, main functions of, 8
Urinary diversion, 53, 104
Urinary frequency, 7
    defined, 19
    delayed voiding and, 61
    detrusor overactivity and, 18
    urodynamic study and assessment of, 45
Urinary incontinence, 8
    causes of, 11–12
    impact of, 29
    medications with side effects contribut-
        ing to, 22t
    nursing home admissions and, 30
    overactive bladder with/without, 20
    potentially treatable causes of, 21
    prevalence of, 10–11
    reversible, management of conditions
        causing, 23t
    urodynamic study and assessment of, 45
Urinary retention, 10, 83
Urinary symptoms, assessment of, 41
Urinary tract, lower, innervation of, 6
Urinary tract infections, 21, 43
    interstitial cystitis and, 16
    overactive bladder and, 25
Urinate, 7
Urine
    backup of, 3
    production of, 2
Urine cytology, 114
Urine leakage, urgency and, 9, 19
Urodynamic study, 24, 44, 106
    defined, 45
    role of, 13, 14

Uroflow, 47
Urogynecologists, 32
Urologists, 33, 112
Urothelium, 2, 25
Uroxatral, 35, 55

V
Vaginal cone, 62
Valsalva maneuver, 12, 13
Vasopressin, nocturia and, 37
Venous stasis, nocturia and, 37
Vesicare, 35, 70, 75–76
    dosing, half-life and metabolism rate of,
        80t
    dosing recommendations for, 94
    side effects with, 86t
Vesicoureteral reflux, 115
Video-urodynamics, 47, 49
Voiding, timed or prophylactic, 56, 60–61
Voiding habits, normal, 7–8
Voiding log/bladder diaries, 41, 41, 59, 60

W
Water pills, 39
Women. See also Females
    antimuscarinics and, 83
    constipation in, 87
    OAB treatment in, 53
    overactive bladder and physical examina-
        tion for, 42
    prevalence of overactive bladder in, 26
    prevalence of urinary incontinence
        among, 11
    rapid pelvic floor contractions and, 56–57
    sacral neuromodulation and, 108
    stress urinary incontinence in, 20
Work life, overactive bladder and, 30

X
Xerostomia (dry mouth)
    common causes of, 90–91
    prevalence of, 90
    treatment of, 91
X-ray tests, hematuria evaluation and, 44

Y
YM 178, 95

DATE DUE